ENDING RACIAL, ETHNIC, AND CULTURAL DISPARITIES IN AMERICAN HEALTH CARE

George C. Halvorson

DEDICATION

*This book is dedicated to the people who died too soon
due to the disparities in their care.*

THANK YOU

Thank you to Dr. Ron Copeland, Dr. Jed Weissberg, Dr. Jack Cochran, Chuck Columbus, Ray Baxter -- and for your great energy and passion on these issues -- Bernard Tyson, for your ongoing support of this work and for your clear, direct, and collective leadership of the Disparity Reduction and Disparity Elimination Efforts and Programs at Kaiser Permanente.

Thanks also to members of Kaiser Permanente chairman's communications team -- including Linda Cruz, Eva De Anda, Victoria Meas, and David Mays -- who worked together to make this book a reality. And thank you to Carolyn Liard, Elaine Riate and Candice Key for supporting me in my day job while I wrote this book.

Contents

CHAPTER TWO

KAISER PERMANENTE SET CARE DISPARITY ELIMINATION GOALS.. 18

CHAPTER THREE

HEALTH CARE AND HEALTH COVERAGE IS CHANGING .. 53

CHAPTER FOUR

CHAPTER FIVE

INTRODUCTION

Disparities kill.

People die every day in this country from health care disparities.

The life expectancy of an African American runs more than four years shorter than the life expectancy of a white American.[1] Four years is a lot of years to lose.

Multiple studies have shown higher rates of several key diseases for both African Americans and Hispanic Americans. There are higher death rates as well for both African Americans and Hispanic Americans when those particular diseases occur.[2]

The risk levels and the death rates for those key diseases are even higher for our Native American people.

It is absolutely clear from the data that differences among the various racial and ethnic groups who make up the American population are very real and highly significant. Many people die every year who would not die if every ethnic and racial group in this country had the same health care outcomes and the same disease levels as our most healthy groups for those same diseases.

A major study of health care disparities that was done by the Institute of Medicine (IOM) in 2003 pointed out both patterns of care and care outcomes that differed significantly from group to group.[3] Some studies included in that report had data about care gaps among the groups that were so significant that they were hard to believe.

In a country that spends 2.8 trillion dollars on care each year[4] -- more money than the total economies of all but five entire nations[5] -- we should not have those kinds of care gaps and we should not experience those kinds of outcome differences among groups of people for our care.

Bias, Biology and Behavior

When you drill down into each of the care gaps that exist, it becomes clear that there are three primary causes for those care differences by group. The three primary causes of those care differences are bias, biology, and behavior.

All three of those causes have an impact. Sometimes the care gaps we see are the result of two or three of those causes working together to jointly impact care, and sometimes the differences we see are the result of just one of those factors. In either case, we need to identify and deal with the relevant causes to reduce the disparities in both care outcomes and consequences.

We need to recognize the unfortunate reality of bias as a cause of disparities. Bias happens. There are multiple cases -- several described in this book -- where care differences among groups of people are simply and directly based on biased decisions made by caregivers. When African American patients and Hispanic patients are both significantly less likely than whites to get a pain reliever when having a heart attack,[6] that pattern of care is clearly based on some level of bias, and it is not based on biology, medical science, or patient behavior. When African Americans and Hispanics and other non-white children with autism who are seen at the same major academic treatment centers are 38 percent to 68 percent less likely than whites to see specialists or subspecialists for nutrition services, gastrointestinal services, neurology or psychiatric services, there is a clear indication of caregiver bias driving those differences in care.[7]

Sometimes the bias is conscious -- and sometimes the bias is unconscious -- but it is never a good thing when bias is part of the care process. We clearly, as a nation, need to address both unconscious and conscious bias as we work to reduce the care gaps and the care disparities we see in America today.

The most recent National Health Care Quality Report, showing care performance levels for 2012, produced this year by the Agency for Healthcare Research and Quality -- described many of those care gaps clearly and pointed out that some of the gaps are actually widening rather than shrinking.[8]

The level of bias that exists in too many instances and that too often causes those gaps in care to happen is not being addressed in any systematic way in this country at this point in time. The bias problem is real -- but there are no plans to make it shrink or disappear.

Biology is also an important factor.

A number of care differences have underlying causes that are clearly biological. The high rates of some cancers for some of our population groups seem to stem primarily from biological issues. The fact that African American women are 47 percent more likely to get multiple sclerosis (MS) than white women seems to be entirely biological -- although it is not impossible that there might be some currently unknown behavioral or environmental issues that are increasing the risk levels of MS in Black women.[9]

One of the best examples of biological differences in risk by group came from a study done by Kaiser Permanente using their electronic medical record database to look at care links and causality factors.

The Kaiser Permanente study showed that when pregnant women have uterine infections during pregnancy, their children are much more likely to have childhood asthma a couple of years later. The data showed that linkage clearly exists.[10]

What makes that important study relevant to this book on care disparities and care differences is that the Kaiser Permanente researchers also used their data to look at the variable impact of that set of infections for children of different racial and ethnic groups.

That particular study showed a significant difference in risk level by group. African American kids were over 90 percent more likely to have childhood asthma if their mothers had that infection. Hispanic children were 70 percent more likely to have childhood asthma if their mothers had that same infection.[11]

White children were 66 percent more likely to have childhood asthma if their mothers had that infection.[12]

So there were clear differences in the disease risk levels for each group of children that were not behavior-based or bias-based in any way for those mothers or for those children.

The most startling finding that resulted from that particular piece of research was for the Asian American mothers and children in the study. Asian American children actually had a zero increase in childhood asthma risk if their mothers had that same infection. There was no additional risk for Asian American children.[13]

All of the expectant mothers from all of the ethnic groups were treated by the same Kaiser Permanente caregivers. They were treated in the same care settings using basically the same care protocols and the same care approaches.

Likewise, all of the children were seen by the same Kaiser Permanente pediatricians in the same care settings using the same basic care approaches.

Bias-based care delivery differences were not the cause of that particular risk factor disparity for those children. Neither was the behavior of the mothers or the behaviors of the children. The risk factor difference for that medical condition was clearly biological... the second B of care differences.

That research is one of the reasons why the Kaiser Permanente organization is now collecting DNA samples from a number of patients who have voluntarily -- with full disclosure and with full written approval -- agreed to have their DNA used for medical research. One goal of that research will be to help discover why those kinds of biological differences in risk levels exist and also to figure out what can be done about them.

In that particular disparity -- the causality factor for the differences by racial and ethnic group relative to who is more susceptible to the disease clearly links back to biology.

BEHAVIOR CREATES RISK DIFFERENCES

Maybe the most important factor to look at relative to difference in care outcomes and care process needs, however, is behavior. We can't change biology -- but we can change behavior. Patient behavior creates major differences in patient risk levels, in disease incidence, and in disease outcomes. To end some of the current care disparities and close the care gaps for some conditions, we need to help patients from each high-risk group successfully achieve healthy behaviors in targeted areas.

What behaviors need to be changed?

Healthy behaviors that improve care outcomes can be as simple as people getting their basic medical tests and having their basic cancer screens done.

Most chronic diseases can be steered to better outcomes with early diagnosis and with ongoing disease monitoring and consistent and continuing treatments.

We know from the data that there are some significant disparities among the racial and ethnic groups in both of those key areas of patient behavior.

This book will show disparities in early diagnosis levels and disparities in care follow-up by patients -- with significant care gaps among the groups of patients in some important areas of care -- like blood pressure control.

Those particular disparities can be ended -- but it takes a clear focus on each group and on each disparity area to have success in eliminating gaps in those areas of care.

Likewise, there are significant differences in cancer survival rates among the racial and ethnic groups that relate back to differences among groups in the early detection of cancer. Again, a major remedy for that particular outcome disparity is to get people from each group to improve their cancer testing levels. Hispanics, for example, are significantly less likely to have colon cancer testing done.[14] That difference in behavior by those patients results in a care gap and in a much higher death rate for the people whose cancer is detected late.

The death rate is significantly higher.

When colon cancer is detected very early in a high quality care setting, the death rate over five years is less than 5 percent. Ninety-five percent of the patients whose cancer was detected early are still alive.[15] When colon cancer is detected late, however, and not discovered until it has reached its more advanced stages -- the death rate for those patients is much higher. Only 12 percent of those late-diagnosed patients are still alive -- on average -- in five years.[16]

Those disparities in care outcomes and those differences in death rates are caused in part by behaviors. The key behavior change that is needed in that instance to end the care gap among groups of people is to get all people to have their colon cancer tests done frequently so that more cancers for every group can be detected at an early stage.

This book describes the impact of those cancer-screening behavioral differences relative to some key cancers. That is an important area of focus on behavior change if we want to reduce some of the major disparities in cancer care outcomes that exist today.

The other area of needed behavior change is even more important. We need people from all groups to have a higher level of healthy behaviors in three key areas. For starters, we need fewer people to smoke. Smoking is the number one cause of lung cancer.[17] There are clear differences in smoking levels among various ethnic and racial groups. We need people from all ethnic groups to stop smoking to reduce the level of that cancer significantly for every group.

The other behaviors we need to change relate to chronic diseases. Chronic diseases drive more than 75 percent of the costs of care in this country today.[18] Chronic diseases are growing at an alarming rate for all ethnic groups. Diabetes, alone, now consumes over 40 percent of the total costs of Medicare, and the number of diabetics in this country is growing to epidemic levels.[19] Diabetes is the fastest growing disease in America and the risk levels for that disease are actually higher for Hispanics, Blacks, and Native Americans than they are for white patients.[20]

The point we need to recognize is this -- diabetes -- and the other key chronic diseases -- are all caused primarily by two basic behaviors. There are some biological risk level differences by group, and there are some neighborhood-related environmental differences that can vary by group -- but the most important behavior-linked risk differences that result in adverse and variable outcomes for those diseases happen at the individual patient level. The overall group level risk differences are increased or decreased hugely for each person by two basic sets of individual patient behaviors.

INACTIVITY AND OBESITY ARE THE TWO KEY DRIVERS FOR CHRONIC DISEASE

It isn't very complicated.

Two key behaviors drive almost all chronic diseases. People can change their risk significantly for those diseases by changing one or two of those behaviors. The two key behaviors that significantly increase risk levels for individual patients are personal inactivity and personal obesity.[21]

We currently have an epidemic of inactivity in this country. More than half of Americans do not achieve the minimum activity levels that are needed to be healthy.[22] Obesity is also at epidemic levels -- with over a third of Americans obese today and a growing number of people clearly on the way to being obese tomorrow.[23]

Both inactivity and obesity significantly increase the risk of our key chronic diseases.[24] Both of those behaviors need to be part of our health strategy if we want to reduce the rate of those key diseases. We need to increase our activity levels, and we need to reduce our weight levels in order to reduce our actual disease levels.

The science that tells us we need to increase our activity levels is very powerful and very encouraging. Walking seems to be an extremely high-value mechanism for improving activity levels. Walking is something we can assist people to do. The human body is clearly made to walk and needs to walk to be healthy. It doesn't take a lot of walking to have a major impact. When we walk 30 minutes a day, 5 or more days each week, the rate of new diabetes cases actually cuts in half.[25]

The diabetes risk level goes down over 60 percent for older Americans when that same level of walking happens for older individuals.[26]

Walking that same amount of time also reduces stroke risk for people by over 40 percent, heart attack risk by over a third, and that level of walking reduces the risk of colon cancer, prostate cancer, and breast cancer by more than a third.[27]

Depression levels go down -- and the functional effectiveness of antidepressant drugs can double -- when people walk that same half-hour a day, five or more days each week.[28]

That point about the need for physical activity and the benefits it creates is highly relevant to this book on care disparities because there are clear risk differences for those diseases by racial and ethnic group, and one of the best ways of making those differences among groups in outcomes and incidence levels disappear is to get people in each group to walk.

Likewise, obesity levels have a huge impact on each of those diseases. Helping people who are obese to eat healthier food and to eat lower quantities of food is clearly also the right thing to do. Both of those efforts to create healthier behaviors need to be linked to the culture and to the group behavior preferences of each set of patients, or they will have a much lower likelihood of success.

Behaviors impact diseases. We need to help the people who are at risk for those diseases to achieve healthy behaviors -- and we need to do that in ways that work in the context and the life reality of each patient and each group member.

We also need to deliver best care to each set of patients when patients from each group incur diseases. We need to eliminate care disparities among groups by significantly improving care for all patients -- and by focusing on the needs of the groups who have a higher risk to keep that risk from disproportionately damaging those groups of patients.

Can that work be done? Can systematic care improvement for those patients and those diseases be done successfully in this country today for each group of people? That is an extremely important question to answer.

THE INSTITUTE OF MEDICINE CALLED FOR BETTER DATA

The highly regarded Institute of Medicine (IOM) taskforce on care disparities a decade ago offered some thoughts about how disparities might be reduced.[29] The report called for better data about disparities -- because the truth is that we really can't deal effectively with disparities until we know exactly what they are and where they exist. The report also called for medical best practices -- with care protocols based on the best science and applied equitably to all groups of patients.

Kaiser Permanente has taken that guidance about both best care practices and the need for better data from that taskforce to heart and has done extensive work to build the database and the data tools that are needed to do that work. Kaiser Permanente has set up internal databases that can now identify care disparities and care differences for the 9 million[30] people who are now served by the Kaiser Permanente care system.

That is a very useful tool kit. It has been the anchor of a significant learning opportunity.

That work wasn't done in small, isolated silent studies.

It was done with a very large population of patients. The population of 9 million people who are served today by the Kaiser Permanente care system is bigger than 40 states and 146 countries.[31] It is also a very diverse set of people -- with over half of the Kaiser Permanente membership coming from one ethnic group or another. There is no majority population inside Kaiser Permanente at this point in time.

So the work that is being done at Kaiser Permanente to deal with differences in care delivery by ethnic group and by race are actually highly and directly relevant to the challenge of dealing with those same issues across all of American health care.

As one example -- one of the programs that was conducted and presented at the most recent annual Kaiser Permanente Diversity Conference was labeled "Designing Culturally Appropriate Tools to Reduce Disparities in Hypertension Control and Colorectal Cancer Screening in Diverse Populations." That work was based on actual care site experience in doing that set of work for those sets of patients in significantly large care settings.

This book deals at a macro level with health care disparities and care differences across America. This book also explains some of the approaches that are currently being used at Kaiser Permanente to improve care for the entire 9 million people and to specifically focus on areas of performance where there are care gaps and care disparities for specific subsets of Kaiser Permanente's 9 million very diverse patients.[32]

THE LEARNINGS SHOULD BE USEFUL FOR OTHER CARE TEAMS

Kaiser Permanente has been on a learning curve for those patients and those issues for several years. Mistakes have been made, challenges have been addressed, learning has improved, and a number of successes have been achieved. This book describes some key points of that learning and shares some of the conclusions that have been reached about dealing with those issues in the actual delivery of care.

Hopefully, this book will be useful for others in this country who are going down similar paths.

Ideally, in future years, other authors inside of Kaiser Permanente will continue to write about this set of programs at Kaiser Permanente. Future books on these topics could benefit everyone in health care.

It is clear that we, as a nation, do need to take steps to reduce health care disparities in America. Those disparities exist and people die because care disparities happen in too many places. Chapter One of this book helps point out how significant many of these national disparities are. Chapter Two deals with some care disparities that exist inside Kaiser Permanente – and it explains what that organization is doing to deal with those issues. Chapter Three deals with the changing health care financing and health care delivery environment in America – identifying ways that the new approaches to care delivery and care financing can reduce disparities. Chapter Four deals with some of the guidelines and strategies that Kaiser Permanente has used to succeed as a prototype accountable care organization (ACO), with a focus on how to use ACO tools to help eliminate care disparities. Chapter Five deals with the ways people align with groups that can result in divisive and problematic care – as well as ways that people can align collectively to make care better and more inclusive.

Overall, it is a complex set of issues. Everything is, in the end, connected to everything else. So taking both a big picture look at the full set of issues and a highly focused look at the learnings of one care system who has focused on those issues is probably the right thing to do at this point in time. This book attempts to do that in a way that is useful to both policymakers and practitioners.

Enjoy the book.

CHAPTER ONE

ENDING RACIAL, ETHNIC, AND CULTURAL DISPARITIES IN AMERICAN HEALTH CARE

Minority patients in America are more likely to wait entire weeks to begin treatment for breast cancer.[33]

Delays in treatment definitely increase the death rate for those minority patients.[34] The screening rates for breast cancer, colorectal cancer, and cervical cancer are also significantly lower for our minority populations.[35] Lower screening rates also increase the death rate -- because late stage cancers are much more difficult to cure than early stage cancers.

Minority patients are also significantly less likely to be diagnosed for depression -- and when minority patients are diagnosed with depression, those patients are significantly less likely to be treated for their depression.[36]

Minority patients whose kidneys fail are significantly less likely than white patients to have been under the care of a kidney specialist prior to the failure of their kidneys.[37]

Black patients are not only significantly less likely to have had specialist care before their kidneys failed, Black patients are also more likely to develop end-stage renal disease (ESRD) than white patients.[38]

Black patients are 1.3 times more likely to have a stroke -- and 3 to 6 times more likely to die from their stroke.[39]

According to the National Health Care Quality Report 2012 -- released in 2013 by the Agency for Healthcare Research and Quality -- health care outcomes, care quality, and access to care are all falling below our national goals in a number of key areas for our entire population.[40] To make matters worse, patient access and success levels for basic treatment in too many areas of basic care are actually lower for minority patients than for white patients in America. The rate of hospital admissions for uncontrolled diabetes, for example, is significantly higher for both Black and Hispanic patients -- compared to white patients -- and the death rate is higher for those patients.[41]

Research has also shown that both Black and Hispanic patients who have heart attacks are less likely than white patients to have received timely treatments[42] and are significantly less likely to have received a painkiller early in the care process.[43] Several studies have shown significantly lower and slower support for pain control for both Hispanic and Black patients. For basic care access, a number of studies have shown that Black and Hispanic patients are less likely to receive coronary artery bypass surgery -- half as likely in one study -- for minority patients whose care needs were a good fit for that surgery.[44]

Multiple studies have shown us that access to health care resources and health care processes is not the same for all patient groups across this country and that Hispanic and Black patients tend to have reduced access to a number of care procedures.

Black, Asian, and Hispanic patients are all also significantly less likely to have a "usual primary care provider" than white patients.[45]

That is a very expensive care shortcoming.

Most care costs and care issues in this country today result from chronic disease. Care outcomes for most chronic diseases tend to be improved when patients have both a primary care provider and easy access to their care team. Both easy access and a "usual" primary care provider were less likely to happen for our Hispanic, Black, and Asian patients.[46]

Diabetes is a problem for all of our ethnic groups. It is now the fastest growing disease in America. The rate of diabetes is higher for our Hispanic and Black populations, and it is much higher for our American Indian populations.[47] Our Alaskan natives are 2.3 times as likely as white adults to be diagnosed with diabetes.[48]

In recent years, African Americans have accounted for a major percentage of the new HIV/AIDS diagnosis. Black patients and Hispanic patients both tend to have a death rate from that disease that is 50 percent or more higher than the death rate for white patients with that disease in most care settings.[49]

Hispanic women have an incidence rate for cancers of the cervix that is 1.38 times the rate for white women, and those patients also have a death rate that is 1.32 times higher than the death rate for white patients with the same disease.[50]

The health problems of our Native American populations are so significant that those issues deserve their own book.

Overall, there are a significant number of examples of care outcomes and care process disparities and differences that are becoming increasingly obvious to the people who are keeping track of the health status of our populations. Data about those care differences is obviously important information to have.

It is clear that we should be taking a long and clear look at our care delivery processes and approaches so we can figure out how we can deliver the right level of care to all patients, regardless of their race, gender, or ethnicity.

THERE ARE DIFFERENCES AND THERE ARE DISPARITIES

When we look at the broad array of available data about comparative care outcomes and care processes, it is clear that there are some significant differences in outcomes and approaches that need to be both understood and responded to by us as a nation if we are truly concerned about the wellbeing of all of our citizens. There are obvious differences in several areas of care. We need to understand why those differences exist. We also need to understand what we should be doing about each of the differences. Where measureable differences exist, we need to look very directly at each of those differences and we need to understand what the relevant factors are for each difference. The differences we see among patient groups are not identical from disease to disease and they are clearly not identical from group to group.

BIOLOGY, BEHAVIOR AND BIAS ALL CREATE CARE DIFFERENCES

The differences -- when we study them closely -- obviously have a variety of causes. Three causes, biology, behavior, and bias -- tend to have the most impact. Biology, behavior and bias all create differences in care delivery and care outcomes. We need to understand which of those differences we see among groups of patients relate to differences in behavior, which relate to differences in biology, and which relate to actual disparities in care delivery, disparities in care access, or are the result of deficient and biased approaches to delivering needed care. All of those causes for care delivery differences exist. We need to know which set of causes are relevant to each disease and each health condition so that we can address each cause in the most effective way.

Bias is clearly a factor we need to understand more clearly and address very directly when it is a cause for the differences in care. Clearly, bias results in a number of care delivery differences that are not based on the medical science and best practices for individual patients.

BEHAVIOR DIFFERENCES ARE IMPORTANT TO UNDERSTAND

Behavior differences are also extremely important differences to understand.

Variations in behavior cause variations in disease risk and disease development. There are several categories of behavior differences.

We very much need to understand which of the differences in care or care delivery are linked to behavior. We clearly need to know when any of the relevant behaviors that cause differences in care outcomes or processes are caregiver behaviors. We also need to know when the behaviors that cause differences in care delivery or care outcomes are patient behaviors.

The answers are not as simple as one might think when first looking at the issue. When Black men who are having a heart attack are half as likely to be given a pain reliever early in the care process,[51] that set of data about caregiver behaviors can indicate the existence of either intentional or unintentional bias causing disparities in care delivery. For that set of differences in care, the behaviors that are relevant to creating the problem are the behaviors of the caregivers whose biased decisions about care create those care disparities.

DISPARITIES ARE INAPPROPRIATE, UNFAIR AND BAD

Disparities, in that sense, are behavioral differences in care delivery that are inappropriate, unfair, and either intentionally or unintentionally biased against a given set of patients. Disparities are bad. Disparities reflect choices that are made -- for one reason or another -- against the self-interest and the best interest of a given set of patients. Denying vaccines to minority patients would be a behavioral disparity. Not testing minority patients for diabetes in order to avoid having to diagnose and treat diabetes for those patients would also be a disparity.

Being less likely to get a pain reliever or a medical procedure for a particular medical condition based on your race or your ethnicity group falls under the heading of care bias disparity. Medication differences of that sort are not a care difference. They are a care disparity.

But the fact that we know that Black women are roughly 70 percent more likely to become diabetic[52] is less the result of care delivery disparities than it is the basic reflection of both biological and behavioral differences for the groups of patients involved. In those instances, we need to address the behavioral differences of the patients -- not the caregivers -- and we also need to reflect and respect the higher levels of biological risk of each group of patients for those diseases in our disease detection, prevention, and treatment programs.

PATIENTS BEHAVIORS AND CARE SYSTEM BEHAVIORS

Behaviors cause some diseases. Other diseases are caused by biology. Black women are 47 percent more likely to get multiple sclerosis (MS).[53] We know that to be true.

If there are any behavioral underpinnings of any kind that might be triggering the higher level of MS that happens for Black women, those causes or those triggers that might increase risk levels for those women for MS are not known. Those differences in the MS rate -- with Black women much more likely to get the disease -- are probably entirely biological instead of behavioral. But for diabetes, the situation is obviously much more complicated. We know for a fact that certain ethnic and racial groups are much more likely to become diabetic than other ethnic and racial groups. There are clearly biological risk factors. But we also know that the biological factors are heavily influenced by patient behaviors. We know that the behaviors of people in each of the higher risk groups can change the risk levels for people in those groups significantly. Diabetes is a great example. We know that individual people in the high-risk groups for that disease can increase the likelihood of personally getting that disease significantly by being physically inert and by being significantly overweight. Behavior is highly relevant for both of those issues. Weight and activity levels are both behavior-based differences that change the risk status for individual people. We know that when people have higher activity levels and when people weigh less, the risk of diabetes drops -- by more than half.[54]

BEHAVIORS TRIGGER DIABETES

Behaviors clearly trigger diabetes. We know that to be true. The science is pretty clear. Both unhealthy eating and unhealthy inactivity trigger that disease. Both of those factors are extremely important. Most people don't understand how important basic activity levels are to diabetes prevention. As noted in the introduction to this book, the correlation between inactivity and diabetes is incredibly strong. A person who walks thirty minutes a day, five days a week is half as likely to become diabetic as a person who does not walk at all or who rarely walks.[55] A person who is inert is much more likely to become diabetic. That is true, regardless of the person's weight. Thin people who are completely inert can actually have a higher chronic disease level than overweight people who walk regularly.[56] Fit beats fat as a risk factor. Both activity and obesity increase the risk of becoming diabetic, however, and you can reduce the number of people who become diabetic with behavior changes that cause people to be consistently active and weigh less.

That set of factors has to be understood in light of the obvious differences in risk for diabetics that exist for different ethnic and racial groups. We obviously need to help our minority populations improve both activity levels and healthy eating levels if we want to stop the epidemic of diabetes from hurting even more people.

That knowledge base about the impact of those behaviors is part of the patient-focused, culturally competent solution set we need to discover, develop and enhance -- so we can deal most effectively with the difference levels that exist for diabetic care for each group of people. We also need to improve our skill sets and knowledge base so we can also significantly reduce the actual care gaps that exist between the various groups for patients who do have diabetes.

Care delivery disparities exist, and they obviously add another level of complexity to the issue. We know that African Americans who have advanced diabetes and kidney failure are, on average, significantly less likely to have seen a kidney specialist before their kidneys failed.[57] Seeing those specialists in a timely manner can actually lead to better care. That better care can help keep a patient's kidneys from failing. A group of people whose kidneys failed because they did not have access to those specialists can fall under the category of care disparity.

But having kidneys fail because the diabetic patient is obese and inert falls more under the category of patient behavior-induced care outcomes rather than outcomes that are being caused by disparities or by bias in care access or care delivery. We will not succeed in our goals of better diabetic outcomes if we focus only on the part of the problem that is caused by care disparities. We need to focus on the overall, targeted outcomes we want for those patients, and then we need to deal with all of the relevant factors -- including biology and behaviors -- as a total package of issues rather than being focused ideologically, functionally, or politically on a subset of the package.

WE CAN REDUCE CARE COSTS BY MAKING CARE BETTER

For us all to be as healthy as we each can be, we need a combination of personal behaviors that can help each of us reduce known risk. We also very much know that we need best care to help cure or minimize the damage that we each suffer when we do have diseases and then need to have those diseases treated. We need to hold the care system to a high level of expected and consistent performance when we each need care.

We need fewer kidneys to fail and we need fewer congestive heart failure patients and asthma patients in the emergency room. We obviously need to coach patients to take the steps needed to reduce the risks of their own health care problems, and we need to help caregivers deliver the right care when health care problems exist.

If we do that entire package well, we can reduce health care costs in the United States by making care better. Many people do not know that result can and should happen. Most of the time, for most medical conditions, better care actually costs less. One percent of the people in this country create 20 percent of all health care costs. Five percent of the population creates nearly 50 percent of all costs.[58] We all know that care costs are not spread evenly across the entire population. We all know that it is much less expensive to prevent a kidney failure than it is to do a kidney transplant. The kidney failure that requires a transplant puts people into that 1-percent high cost category that consumes so many of our health care dollars. It is much better to do interventions with several categories of patients to help keep those patients out of that 1-percent category. It is particularly important to do those interventions for our minority patients who the reports all show are much more likely to have their kidneys fail and then die from that disease.

We need to look at real cost numbers as we build our plans to improve care in America for all groups of people. As noted earlier, roughly 70 percent of the costs of care in this country relate to chronic conditions -- like diabetes, asthma, and congestive heart failure.[59] The burden of those diseases also all tend to fall more heavily on our minority patient populations. That burden is exacerbated for many of our minority patients by the fact that the current lack of care delivery resources that are available for many of our minority patients makes early intervention for far too many of those patients relative to those key diseases much less likely to happen. So we have disparities in the availability of care resources for groups of people.

Insurance Disparities Exist as Well

We also face some significant intergroup disparities relative to health insurance today.

Health insurance disparities clearly exist.

The current lack of health insurance for far too many minority Americans is a significant disparity in its own right. As we look at areas where we can differentiate disparities from differences, health insurance has long been an area of significant -- and functionally relevant -- disparity. Over half of the uninsured people in this country today are minority.[60] In some very diverse states -- like California -- over 75 percent of the uninsured people are minority.[61] There is a clear and functional relationship between being insured and getting needed care for many patients. Not having insurance coverage to pay for care creates significant disparities for some people relative to having access to care -- particularly access to the levels of primary care where both early interventions and provider coached, patient-focused, patient-targeted behavior changes can significantly reduce the burden of those diseases for specific patients and groups of patients.

The Health Reform Law Is Intended to Reduce Insurance Disparities

That particular historical disparity relative to a high percentage of American minorities being uninsured will be significantly alleviated for many people at the beginning of next year. Those disparities will shrink for many people on January 1 because the new Affordable Care Act has an aggressive and extensive program that will extend coverage to many of our poorest Americans.

Medicaid will be significantly expanded in many settings. Those Medicaid expansions will help a lot with the current disparities problem in those states that decide to expand Medicaid. Our current national Medicaid program covers many of our poorest citizens now -- but Medicaid is not a comprehensive program today for all poor Americans.

People of color are disproportionately likely to continue to face coverage gaps due to state decisions not to expand Medicaid. In states that do not expand Medicaid, poor, uninsured adults will not gain a new coverage option and likely remain uninsured. People of color make up the majority of uninsured individuals with incomes below the Medicaid expansion limit in states that are not moving forward with the expansion at this time.[62] Moreover, nearly half of all uninsured people of color with incomes below the Medicaid expansion limit reside in states that are not currently moving forward with the expansion.[63] Disparities in coverage and care are likely to persist in states that do not expand Medicaid due to continued coverage gaps.

The new Medicaid program that will begin next year in most states will cover all citizens who are just above and below the official federal poverty level. It isn't entirely clear yet how many states will expand their Medicaid programs at this point. The current coverage disparities issue will not be significantly reduced in those states that do not expand Medicaid. In most of the states where the planned Medicaid expansion will happen, however, the majority of the newly enrolled Medicaid-eligible people will be minority patients, and that will directly reduce the insurance coverage disparity trends.

THE NEW INSURANCE EXCHANGES WILL BENEFIT LOW INCOME PEOPLE AS WELL

As noted above, not all states will expand Medicaid. All states will, however, put in place new health insurance "exchange" markets for individual insurance coverage. Those new "exchanges" will provide access to subsidized coverage for low income people in all states. In some states, the new subsidized insurance market will supplement the expanded Medicaid programs. In other states,

Medicaid will not expand, and the new exchanges will be the only program that helps reduce the current coverage disparity gaps. All states will have the new exchanges in place, however, and the exchanges will all provide subsidies for lower income people who decide to buy private health insurance through the exchanges. Those exchanges will be a very different way of buying individual health insurance.

The new insurance exchanges will offer competing private health plans as choices to all Americans who want to directly buy health insurance. In the past, people who wanted to buy individual insurance coverage in this country almost always needed to pass a health screen that was set up by each of the health insurance companies. The new law eliminates those health screens for the purchase of individual health insurance. There will be no health screens used by insurers in the new exchanges. Everyone in this country who wants to buy individual health insurance will now be able to buy that insurance, regardless of their current or past health status. The disparity issues that exist today for health insurance coverage will be helped significantly by the new exchanges because low income people who decide to buy their own health insurance through their local exchange will receive a subsidy from the government to make their premiums more affordable. A slight majority of the low income uninsured people who will have an opportunity to buy that subsidized insurance in most states will be from our minority populations.

THE PREMIUM SUBSIDIES FOR LOWER INCOME PEOPLE WILL BE SIGNIFICANT

The premium subsidies available in the exchanges will be significant. They will pay most of the premiums for the lowest income people who buy coverage in the exchange. That subsidy approach will, of course, make premiums much more affordable for many low income people.

That process and that program are not yet in place. The exchanges are being built, however, for January 1 effective dates. When they are in place, some of the current disparities that exist in insurance coverage by race and ethnicity should be reduced.

It's not known yet how many low income people will enroll in the exchanges. The actual number of people who will be eligible for the expanded Medicaid coverage also isn't entirely clear yet -- but the numbers in both programs will be significant, and that new coverage agenda clearly should help narrow the gap and reduce the number of people who will face the disparity of being uninsured.

GUARANTEED ACCESS TO INSURANCE DOES NOT CREATE GUARANTEED ACCESS TO CARE

Those two insurance coverage expansion programs will not deal in any way with roughly 10 million currently uninsured people who are undocumented non-citizens.[64] But the newly subsidized insurance coverage and the major new Medicaid expansion could make a significant reduction in the number of uninsured citizens. Minority enrollment in those programs will help people get guaranteed access to insurance coverage -- but not, necessarily, guaranteed access to actual health care.

ACCESS TO COVERAGE DOESN'T CREATE ACCESS TO CARE

Access to actual care will not be guaranteed by the fact that people have become insured. Access to coverage does not guarantee access to care. The newly insured people will still need to find care sites and caregivers. In a number of areas, the number of care sites that will be available to the newly insured people may well be inadequate.

So ending coverage disparities would not end care disparities -- but reducing those disparities in insurance will significantly give the country a much better chance of eliminating disparities in care.

SOME CARE GAPS ARE WIDENING

That set of circumstances and those changes in who will be insured next year in America obviously raises an interesting and important set of questions for us all -- in addition to creating some important opportunities. We need to take advantage of the opportunities to help end disparities in care. Disparities will continue to exist. So will differences in care delivery and health status. The data that shows significant differences in care levels, disease burdens and care outcomes between various racial and ethnic groups is both clear and compelling. Those differences and disparities truly exist, and they will continue to exist. As noted earlier, The National Health Care Quality Report for 2012 -- released this year -- said that the care gaps between some of the groups in some key areas of care delivery are widening rather than narrowing.[65]

If some care gaps are widening -- and if we really do believe as a nation that we should have a health care strategy, infrastructure, and an overall collective commitment to having the right care for each segment of our population -- then we need to look to see what strategies we can put in place to help us meet our overall goals of better care for all Americans.

The truth is we can't just make isolated changes in some areas of care delivery and hope to either reduce care disparities or improve care.

We need to make some significant changes in the way we deliver care to fully achieve those goals.

WE NEED BETTER SYSTEMS, APPROACHES, AND TOOLS

This is actually a very good time for us to make some meaningful changes in the way we deliver care. That very powerful and well-researched IOM report that was written in 2003 about the issues we face as a country relative to care disparities said at that point in time that we need to make some significant changes in the systems, approaches, and tools we use to support care in order to create real improvement relative to many areas of care disparities.[66] The experts who created that 2003 report said we need better data, we need data by ethnic groups, we need data about a wider range of care delivery functions and areas, and we need better care support tools. They said we needed medical best practices, and we need those best practices consistently applied across all groups. The authors of that pioneering and insightful 2003 report were entirely correct. We do need some better tools, and we very much need significantly better and timelier data to deal effectively with most care disparities and most care improvement issues. Fortunately, we are currently in a time of great change and innovation for care delivery, and it is possible now -- for the first time in the history of care delivery -- to make some real changes that can make care better, more accessible, more affordable, and even more equitable for the patients of this country. This is a good time to improve care.

THE SCIENCE AND PRACTICE OF CARE IS GETTING BETTER

The science of care is actually getting continuously better. The tool kits that are being used to support care delivery are getting much better. Electronic medical records, remote monitoring tools, and new electronic connectivity tools are all offering us new ways of thinking about care delivery that were not available to us just a few years ago. Electronic medical records are now giving us much better data about both individual patient care and about effective population care. We now can keep track of both patients and populations of patients in much more effective ways. We are currently poised at the edge of a possible revolution in both care connectivity and care improvement.

This is a very exciting time for care delivery -- and the good news for the issue of care disparities is that the entire new array of tools and services can and should be used to help us deal more effectively with the issues that we now face relative to both care disparities and care differences in American health care. Progress in all of those areas is now possible in ways that real progress functionality could not happen back in 2003 when that particular report was written. Those authors were ahead of their time -- but their dream can be actualized today. That isn't a hypothetical, speculative, or wishfully optimistic statement about the possibility of care improvement today. That statement about the possibility of real progress today is a belief that is based on some real-world, site-specific applications of several of those tools over the past couple of years in ways that have helped caregivers accomplish those exact goals and do it in a systematic, process-supported care environment.

The people who wrote that very powerful report said that care delivery would need better data, information flows that could be delineated to identify and focus on performance differences by race and ethnicity, and a higher dependence on medical best practices with best practices consistently applied for all people and all groups of patients. Those thinkers were entirely correct. That approach does work. The good news today is that we now have a real-world experiment that involves 9 million very diverse people who are being served today with the basic care support tool kits that were envisioned in the 2003 report.

That diverse population is the 9 million people who are now served by the Kaiser Permanente care system.[67] As the introduction to this book pointed out, that care system has made an explicit and direct commitment to ending disparities in care delivery for the 9 million people it serves, and it is using some of the very tools that were described and recommended by the 2003 IOM report on health care disparities to do that work.

Kaiser Permanente has done some learning about those tools over the past several years. One learning is that it isn't enough to simply put the tools in place and hope that care gets better. Electronic medical records on their own and by themselves cure nothing. They aren't magic. They are tools.

Those tools need to be used, and they need to be used well -- but when that happens, disparities can be reduced, and the care differences that still exist can be care differences that are appropriate to the patient and functionally represent best care.

That targeted disparity-reduction work that has been done over the past several years at Kaiser Permanente needs to be better understood. That is the purpose of the next portion of this book.

Care disparities and differences exist in the U.S. We all know that to be true. People die every day because those disparities happen. It should be unacceptable to us as a nation to continue to have those huge differences in care outcomes -- and a four-year difference in the lifespan of people based on their race or ethnic group should not be acceptable to us as a country.

We need to look at the ways we can improve care for everyone and at the ways we can reduce disparities in care delivery and key outcomes. Care gaps should not happen.

CHAPTER TWO

===

KAISER PERMANENTE SET CARE DISPARITY ELIMINATION GOALS

As the last chapter noted and as the introduction to this book pointed out, a real-world test of the 2003 disparity report recommendations to use a combination of group-specific data, focused care support tools, and medical best practices that are aimed specifically at reducing disparities in care is happening today at Kaiser Permanente. Kaiser Permanente is a health care delivery and financing organization that serves more than 9 million people.[68] The people who are served by Kaiser Permanente constitute one of the most diverse patient populations in America. The Kaiser Permanente membership is currently more than half minority.[69] In the rest of the country, about 30 percent of all patients today are from minority groups.[70] More than half of the patients who get care in the Kaiser Permanente care system come from one minority group or another. So Kaiser Permanente is not only a useful setting for looking at care trends today, Kaiser Permanente already looks like the rest of America will look in a decade or two. Kaiser Permanente has already recognized a broad range of implications that can result from a high level of patient diversity, and the care teams have worked both strategically and functionally to directly address multiple issues that relate to care differences and to disparities in care delivery. The care teams at Kaiser Permanente have been able to do that work with a robust set of care support tools. The new databases and tool kits also reflect the new tool kits that will be available relatively soon to support care in other care sites across the country.

So Kaiser Permanente is a diverse care system serving a very diverse set of patients and doing that work using a set of computerized care support tools that are likely to be the next generation of care support tools. In that context, addressing care disparities has been a high priority.

A wide range of issues relating to care disparities, care differences, and various methods of dealing with delivery processes and delivery issues for various groups of people have been the focus of very serious thinking and careful planning at Kaiser Permanente. That has been true for the past several years. This has been an important and pioneering area of work for care delivery. That will be a useful model and experiment for American care sites. That work has been a high-value learning experience for the Kaiser Permanente care teams who do that work. It has been very useful and educational to record, monitor, and utilize the results. Kaiser Permanente has been very directly addressing the multiple challenges and opportunities that are presented by a complex and changing care environment and a diverse set of patients.

Why did Kaiser Permanente do that work?

Kaiser Permanente is functionally accountable for both the care and the health of more than 9 million people. That is obviously a major and large-scale commitment to population health. The Kaiser Permanente organization decided to set an official and very specific goal of eliminating internal care disparities for the 9 million people who are served by that organization several years ago. The Kaiser Permanente care teams have been using their resources, tool kits, and a wide of array of care expertise to accomplish that goal.

ADDRESSING DISPARITIES HAS BEEN A PROCESS OF CONTINUOUS LEARNING

That work has been a process of continuous learning. As a result of that commitment and that agenda, Kaiser Permanente now has had several years of learning, experimentation, and process improvement operational rollouts that are worth describing, sharing, and explaining to the rest of the health care world at this point in time.

A number of policy experts who have focused over the years on various aspects of care- disparity issues have tended to look at the overarching issues of care differences and at care disparities from a theoretical, academic, high level, often only vaguely functional macro policy perspective. That kind of macro analysis and theoretical thinking is good work to do – but those efforts usually do not change the actual delivery of care in any functional care site. Kaiser Permanente, by contrast, has looked at those same sets of issues very explicitly and very directly from the highly immediate and very practical perspective of being – at its core – an operational care delivery organization and a functional infrastructure of care. That work that is being done on those care disparity and core differences issues at Kaiser Permanente in the context of that care infrastructure may well be somewhat useful to other caregivers across the countries who are actually wrestling with those same sorts of issues from a functional and operational perspective.

KAISER PERMANENTE IS A LARGE-SCALE MICROCOSM

The rest of the country is becoming more diverse. That fact of our increasing diversity was cited again as a key issue for us all to think about in the newest federal study of care gaps in this country -- The National Health Care Quality Report 2012.[71] That study suggested that our increasing diversity as a nation should call for us to increase our focus on eliminating intergroup disparities in care. As noted above, Kaiser Permanente already has over half of its patient population from one minority group or another and is dealing with those issues now.

In addition to having a diverse set of patients, Kaiser Permanente is serving all of those diverse people in the functional context of being a basically self-contained care and financing system. This is an important fact to understand because it creates great opportunities for structured care improvement processes. Kaiser Permanente doesn't just "insure" care. Kaiser Permanente actually delivers care -- from its own internal, vertically integrated care system. It is very important to understand the pure functional fact that Kaiser Permanente is a somewhat unique care delivery organization. Kaiser Permanente is, in fact, an almost unique combination of care delivery and care financing. Kaiser Permanente enrolls those roughly 9 million members in a health plan, and then provides care to those 9 million people primarily through care delivery sites that are owned and operated by Kaiser Permanente.[72]

THE KAISER PERMANENTE WORKFORCE IS 58 PERCENT MINORITY

Kaiser Permanente has about 180,000 internal employees -- with over 160,000 of the Kaiser Permanente people involved in delivering care or supporting the people who deliver care.[73] It is also important to note that the workforce at Kaiser Permanente is even more diverse than the patient base.

Roughly, 58 percent of the people who are working at Kaiser Permanente today come from one minority group or another.[74] In other words, the workforce at Kaiser Permanente today looks a lot like the total workforce of America will look like in relatively a few years. A major workforce change will actually happen relatively quickly for the rest of America because a majority of the young people who will be entering the American workforce over the next few years will be coming from one minority group or another. Kaiser Permanente has achieved that level of minority workforce already and can also serve as a template and a model for the impact of diversity on the care delivery workforce.

Kaiser Permanente is not a small organization. That fact also makes this set of work relevant. The disparity-reduction and gap-closure work that is being done at Kaiser Permanente has not been done in isolated and small care sites. Kaiser Permanente is actually one of the larger hospital systems in the country -- with 38 licensed hospitals.[75] It is also one of the larger care site owners in the world -- with roughly 630 owned and operated care sites.[76]

Two of the seven Permanente Medical Groups are the largest private medical groups in the world.[77]

Kaiser Permanente owns labs, pharmacies, imaging centers, and multiple other categories of care sites. The Kaiser Permanente laboratory system runs roughly 81,000 tests every day[78] -- and the pharmacy system fills roughly 200,000 prescriptions a day.[79]

It was noted earlier that Kaiser Permanente serves more people as a care system than 40 states and 146 countries.[80] Total revenues at Kaiser Permanente exceed $50 billion a year.[81] That money is almost entirely collected in monthly premium payments from each patient. Collecting money through premiums is a very different cash flow approach than the cash flow used by most other care organizations in America. Most other care sites sell care by the piece -- not by the package. The standard piecework business model for American health care involves having all revenue for each care site collected from a fee schedule -- with separate bills charged by each care site to each patient for each piece of care. The rest of health care tends to use that very basic piecework payment model, and most care sites sell care entirely and only by the piece. Kaiser Permanente primarily uses a lump sum cash flow model, and the cash flow at Kaiser Permanente is not based on selling pieces of care.

So overall, Kaiser Permanente is large and basically self-contained as a care delivery infrastructure -- and Kaiser Permanente has a revenue stream that buys entire packages of care for groups of patients rather than just having individual patients paying for individual pieces of care. The Kaiser Permanente model may also be the future model for care financing. Health care reform efforts for the country are attempting in many ways to create a similar cash flow model for other care sites. Those issues and those efforts are addressed more directly in the next chapter of this book. The reality today is that the integrated care delivery structure and the packages of care and cash payment cash flow approach has allowed Kaiser Permanente to put in place an extensive set of care tools that do not exist in most other care settings.

That new tool kit includes what is probably the largest electronic medical record support system in the world as a care support tool for its caregivers. Kaiser Permanente now has an electronic medical record in place for all 9 million of its patients.

That massive electronic health record care support system supports the function of allowing each doctor to have all of the medical information about each of their patients available to the doctor in real time when the information about each patient is needed by the doctor at the point of care. The rest of American health care is currently moving in basically that same direction -- with the goal of having electronic data about each patient in place in each care site in this country relatively soon. Significant progress is being made in that regard in many American care sites. Care information about each patient is being computerized in a rapidly growing number of care settings across the country. Kaiser Permanente has already achieved that foundational, operational, and functional status as a fully computerized care system, and the care team uses those tools to support care delivery today. That has also been an important part of the learning process. Kaiser Permanente is both developing and refining the operational use of that new information resource, and that new care-support tool kit in an internal process of continuous improvement.

TOP QUALITY SCORES

In total, Kaiser Permanente has built a very useful tool kit for its caregivers that really does improve care delivery. The work that has been done to date to help improve care delivery using those new tools has resulted in dozens of health care quality scores where the highest scores in the entire country -- and, therefore, probably the highest scores in the entire world -- are now at Kaiser Permanente.

That information about Kaiser Permanente and that new care support electronic tool kit that is being used at Kaiser Permanente is relevant to this book about health care disparities, and it is relevant to the differences in care that exist today among groups of people in this country because the Kaiser Permanente experiment proves that the 2003 IOM taskforce authors were correct about the need for tools to end disparities. The IOM disparity team identified some key tools that they believed would be needed to reduce disparities in care. Kaiser Permanente has invested more than $4 billion to put those tools in place and to learn how to use them.[82]

In other words, the process of systems rollout at Kaiser Permanente has shown that the IOM authors were correct, and that we do need the bulk of those tools to be in place in order to reduce many of the care gaps that exist in care delivery in this country. We can't reduce the gaps in care without care improvement tools, and when those tools are in place, care can be improved.

The IOM report called for better tracking of care data by race and ethnicity.

Kaiser Permanente is doing exactly that -- recording care delivery and care performance data by race and ethnicity. The charts shown later in this chapter show the care levels for various ethnic and racial groups of patients, and that data shows some performance gaps among patients of different races and ethnicities that were not expected. The data showed that gaps in care outcomes and processes can happen even in a fully integrated care delivery infrastructure that is committed to having no care gaps of any kind.

KAISER PERMANENTE IS HIGHLY DIVERSE – AT EVERY LEVEL

It was particularly surprising to learn about those gaps because there is no majority group today inside Kaiser Permanente for the Kaiser Permanente staff and care team. Fifty-eight percent of the caregivers and the workers today and more than half of the patients at Kaiser Permanente are minority.[83]

Kaiser Permanente has a diverse staff, a diverse patient base, and Kaiser Permanente also has a very diverse senior leadership group. That leadership diversity is also an important point to mention in discussing the disparity issues that were discovered when the data was reviewed.

There are a number of organizations in this country that currently have a diverse overall workforce. The pattern of diversity in most companies is that they are fairly diverse at the very front level of the workforce, but they are increasingly less diverse when you get to the senior leadership levels. The corporate board rooms of America, for example, tend to be overwhelmingly white and overwhelmingly male. So are the executive suites of most major American companies.

That isn't the pattern at Kaiser Permanente.

Last year, there were eight regional presidents at Kaiser Permanente who were responsible for the eight health plan regions. Only two of the eight presidents were white males. Kaiser Permanente had three group presidents. None were white males. The chief operating officer last year was African American, and the chief financial officer was a woman.[84] As was the controller. The board of directors last year was also only 40 percent white male.[85] In a world where the board of directors of those organizations that have more than $50 billion in annual revenue tend not to be very diverse -- Kaiser Permanente has a highly diverse board, a diverse leadership team, a diverse workforce, a diverse patient base, and a diverse membership. As noted earlier, that level of diversity makes Kaiser Permanente almost a perfect template and setting to look at some of the key issues that relate to growing levels of diversity in American health care and in America as a nation.

THAT DIVERSE ORGANIZATION RATES NUMBER ONE IN MULTIPLE PERFORMANCE AREAS

How well does that very diverse organization function and perform compared to the rest of American health care on various categories of service and care quality? Some people in other organizations have expressed concern about the impact of growing diversity on the performance levels for their organizations. The opposite result has been the reality at Kaiser Permanente. That very diverse blend of people in the Kaiser Permanente workforce has earned some important quality and service recognitions for both caregivers and health plans. The care and service levels at Kaiser Permanente often rate at the number-one level for the entire country.

As one example, Medicare officially rated all health plans in America last year using 55 measures of quality and service. Medicare used that 55 data-based measure set to judge all 563 Medicare health plans across the country on a scale of one star to five stars.[86] The plans with the best quality and the best service scores in the country were awarded five stars by Medicare. The worst plans in the country received one star.

Only 11 health plans in the entire country were awarded all five stars by Medicare.[87] Kaiser Permanente had all eight regions included in that scoring system. Seven of the eight Kaiser Permanente regions earned all five stars and the eighth region earned four point five stars.[88] Likewise -- J.D. Power and Associates rated all commercial health plans for their performance levels last year. For each of the larger Kaiser Permanente regions, J.D. Power and Associates rated the Kaiser Permanente plans number one in service.[89]

The Leapfrog Group is a national organization that does an overall safety rating of American hospitals. The Leapfrog group rates hospitals from A to F, based on their relative safety.[90] Thirty-six of the thirty-eight Kaiser Permanente hospitals were given A ratings. The other two hospitals received B ratings.[91]

The Joint Commission has adopted a couple of Kaiser Permanente care innovations as best practices, and The Commission rates Kaiser Permanente hospitals highly.[92]

Several other awards for quality, service, creativity, and functionality are listed in the appendix to this book. The top scores that were given by the Healthcare Information and Management Systems Society (HIMSS) annual review of hospitals computerization success across the country went to 66 out of 4,000 total U.S.

hospitals. Kaiser Permanente hospitals made up 36 of the 66 top HIMSS-rated hospitals.[93] Kaiser Permanente is the only health care organization to be recognized with the top Uptime Award for its computer systems availability[94] -- and a major Kaiser Permanente data processing site is the only healthcare LEED Platinum-certified data site in the entire country.[95]

Satmetrix rated Kaiser Permanente as having the most credible brand among its members of any major health plan in the country.[96]

So the answer about the relative performance levels that are being achieved by the highly diverse Kaiser Permanente organization is that a highly diverse health plan and care system with a highly diverse staff, a highly diverse membership, a highly diverse leadership, and a highly diverse patient base has ended up being recognized repeatedly as being among the very top performers for the entire nation in multiple objective competitive scoring situations for both care quality and care and health plan service levels.

Diversity is clearly an asset and a strength for Kaiser Permanente performance. In that context, it is entirely understandable that the care team leadership at Kaiser Permanente set the goal several years ago of not having any disparities in care delivery outcome levels for any groups of its patients.

To achieve that goal -- and to clearly focus on any health care differences and disparities that might exist -- Kaiser Permanente very strategically added ethnic and racial group categories to its internal reporting for multiple issues of quality and service. Kaiser Permanente keeps track of about 75 ethnic and racial categories in its recordkeeping.[97] Adding that data to the electronic health record system was a very important thing to do. Kaiser Permanente isn't limited to looking at just the macro, overall performance levels for major areas of care delivery. That macro and blended performance data for all patients is how most care systems and health plans record data. That blended data approach is functionally insufficient to identify real care differences and real care disparities and to identify exactly where they are occurring. More detailed data is needed. Kaiser Permanente accepted that reality and that need for more group-based data and made the system changes that were needed to support that work. Kaiser Permanente now measures both overall performance in those areas as an organization and measures many areas of performance in targeted areas of care based on race and ethnicity. That is pioneering work. It may be unique. That set of data differentials has proven to be an extremely useful and highly educational thing to do. Without that data, Kaiser Permanente could not identify disparities and could not deal effectively with them.

KAISER PERMANENTE COLLECTS PERFORMANCE DATA BY RACE AND ETHNICITY

That work very much resembles the approach to data collection that was suggested by the 2003 IOM report on care disparities. That work has been even more useful than many people suspected it might be when the new data sets were built into the database. Issues like blood pressure control -- where the Kaiser Permanente overall quality scores for the entire population of patients have led the entire country -- were looked at both as an overall score for all Kaiser Permanente patients and as separate performance levels for each group of patients. Key data for each Kaiser Permanente site was collected and reviewed for each major patient group. That data review looked, for example, at blood pressure control for white patients, Black patients, Asian patients, and Hispanic patients. That is a very useful way to look at that set of data -- and it was not possible to do that level of data review until relatively recently. The ability to do that work, to track, record, and report performance by group had to be built into both the electronic medical record database and into the reporting system. That work was done deliberately, intentionally, systematically, skillfully, consistently, and very carefully by Kaiser Permanente.

With data on more than 75 racial and ethnic groups, it was useful to group the datasets into a couple of key categories. Those summary categories were, not coincidentally, the same basic categories used by the U.S. government to do some of its key data reporting.

RACE AND ETHNICITY PERFORMANCE DATA

Almost no one else who delivers volumes of care in this country has that capability to do that level of reporting — and no one in private health care has that kind of information for 9 million patients. That functionality is now being used to identify how well Kaiser Permanente is doing on a number of key performance measures for each of those groups of patients.

THAT DATA HAS BEEN A GOLD MINE FOR RESEARCH

The ability that was set up by Kaiser Permanente to look at care data by race and ethnicity has been a gold mine for medical research as well as for functional improvement. As one example of a recent research gold nugget, the standard belief in health care has long been that Black women were less likely to have Multiple Sclerosis (MS). That long-standing belief is built into many care textbooks. That belief is, in fact, entirely wrong. Medical science now knows the old belief was wrong because Kaiser Permanente has now been able to look at real data for millions of people to see who was really at risk for that disease. The old belief was "MS is primarily a disease of Northern Europeans." The researchers at Kaiser Permanente looked at data for millions of diverse patients and discovered that Black women are actually 47 percent more likely to have MS.[98] It took the new electronic Kaiser Permanente database to uncover that piece of key information about actual risk levels by group. That piece of research is now creating a new core belief about that disease, and it is likely to help many caregivers make accurate diagnoses much earlier with Black patients.

Another important study done with the new database looked at the impact of uterine infections during pregnancy on subsequent asthma risk for children. That study was mentioned in the introduction to this book. The study discovered that higher asthma risk exists for those children -- and that the risk varies by group. As noted earlier, the data showed that Black children have a 90 percent higher asthma risk if their mothers had that infection during pregnancy. Hispanic children have a 70 percent higher risk. White children have a 66 percent higher risk. And Asian American children, the researchers learned, have no additional risk of any kind. Zero.[99]

CHART – 2.1

FOR ILLUSTRATIVE PURPOSES ONLY

Uterine Infection During Pregnancy Linked to Asthma

African Americans	**98%**	increase
Hispanics	**70%**	increase
Caucasians	**66%**	increase
Asian/Pacific Islanders	**0%**	increase

Source: Archives of Pediatric and Adolescent Medicine

That new electronic database is allowing some extremely important scientific learning to happen.

Kaiser Permanente is actually an almost perfect setting to do that kind of research into multiple intergroup issues. It is an almost perfect research site for those kinds of studies because all of the patients from every group at Kaiser Permanente receive their care at the same care sites from the same caregivers. For the mothers in the study that showed the link between uterine infections and childhood asthma, all of the care for all of the mothers and all of the care for all of the kids came from the same care teams and the same care sites. The care protocols used for our patients were fundamentally the same. Also, all of the patients in the Kaiser Permanente database tend to have basically the same insurance coverage. That fact creates basically the same financial reality for care costs for all patients as the financial reality relative to those costs for every other patient who is served by those care sites and those caregivers. In many other medical research circumstances and settings, the patients who are being studied in the research projects who do come from various ethnic groups often can be patients who are using different care sites, different care teams, and they can also very easily be patients who have very different insurance coverage and provider reimbursement realities. At Kaiser Permanente -- for all practical purposes -- the only significant variable that changes for each of the studies of care differences by race and ethnicity is literally the race and ethnicity of the patient. That is a wonderful data environment for doing important medical research on those issues.

The most useful short-term use of that data, however, was to see what actual performance data showed relative to care differences and care disparities when Kaiser Permanente looked at the care performance for multiple quality measures by race and ethnic group.

THE RESULTS WERE NOT IDENTICAL BY RACE AND ETHNICITY

Some of the researchers who looked at the first data runs about relative care performance were shocked. Some people believed that the care results at Kaiser Permanente would be close to identical for every group. They expected almost identical care outcomes and care processes exactly because all of the patients were going to the same care sites, had the same health coverage, and were seeing the same doctors and care teams. The expectation was that all of that functional care delivery consistency would create an equivalent performance consistency for each group of patients. When the actual performance data was reported, however, it was clear that differences among groups existed. Some of the differences were significant. That was an extremely important thing to learn. The performance data variations that existed inside Kaiser Permanente by race and ethnicity showed that even inside a closed care system with the same basic benefit plans for every patient, there can be significant differences in care outcomes and in care performance levels among various ethnic and racial groups. It turned out that there were some entirely unintentional care outcome differences, and it turned out that some care delivery modifications were actually needed to bring all care to the same care level set as the goal of complete equity that was set by the Kaiser Permanente care leaders.

As so often happens for health care quality issues, real data dislodged prior expectations about care performance levels. That learning and that ability to look at real-time data about those issues coupled with the ability to work to correct any problems that might exist makes the Kaiser Permanente experience and learnings on those issues very relevant to this book about health care disparities and differences and to people who are doing health care policy work relative to care disparities and differences.

ACTUAL RESULTS VARIED BY RACE AND GROUP

The next chart shows the actual results by ethnic group inside Kaiser Permanente for the control of blood pressure. Blood pressure control is an extremely important medical goal for the Kaiser Permanente care system. High blood pressure can create heart damage and strokes. Kaiser Permanente has set a major goal for the overall program and care infrastructure of helping patients keep their blood pressure under control. Multiple tools are being used by the Kaiser Permanente care teams to support that goal. The electronic medical record tool kit at Kaiser Permanente and various care reminder support systems are all being used to encourage both caregivers and patients to manage each patient's blood pressure levels.

CHART – 2.2

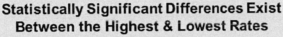

**Statistically Significant Differences Exist
Between the Highest & Lowest Rates**

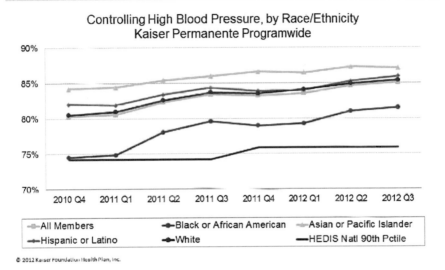

Controlling High Blood Pressure, by Race/Ethnicity
Kaiser Permanente Programwide

© 2012 Kaiser Foundation Health Plan, Inc.

As you can see from that blood pressure chart, the results by ethnic group and by race were not identical. The actual performance data showed that there was a clear difference relative to the Kaiser Permanente success levels on blood pressure control for Black patients compared to white patients, Hispanic patients, and Asian patients.

That finding triggered some significant internal concern. That data also focused intellectual energy in multiple ways for members of the Kaiser Permanente care team. As noted earlier, it was clearly not acceptable to the Kaiser Permanente care team to have internal differences among groups and to have measurable gaps in performance by race or ethnicity group for any key areas of care performance. Those same types of comparative process reports that showed those results for blood pressure health were run for multiple performance areas. Other areas of performance generally had similar results -- with care gaps of some kind in every intergroup comparative performance report. The overall data relative to all performance gaps showed that those gaps were not limited to blood pressure control. The data showed similar patterns involving similar gaps in success levels for several other key quality measures. As described below, the variation in performance lines by race and ethnic group on several other performance charts looked a lot like the separate lines by group on this blood control pressure chart.

THE RED LINE IS 90 PERCENT FOR THE REST OF THE COUNTRY

It is useful to put this particular set of data into perspective.

For blood pressure data shown on this chart, the lower solid red line that is shown as the bottom line on the performance chart actually is an external data-point line. The data on that line includes current performance data from other care sites. That red performance line on the chart is not a Kaiser Permanente performance level. That red line is actually the 90th percentile for all of the other health plans in America who also measure performance on this particular quality metric.

As you can see, even though the Black patients at Kaiser Permanente were doing less well on blood pressure control than the white, Asian, or Hispanic patients at Kaiser Permanente, those Black patients at Kaiser Permanente were doing better on blood pressure control than 90 percent of all of the other patients in all of the other care sites across America who report their performance on that particular measure.

That fact made the lower performance scores for that set of patients inside Kaiser Permanente slightly more tolerable -- but the differences in results and the performance gap between the Black patients and other groups of patients were still not acceptable to the Kaiser

Permanente care team. Care leaders looked at those performance gap numbers and decided that the overall care team needed to figure out how to narrow or eliminate those gaps. That care improvement work and that data analyses were done at a very local level as well as at our overall level. The performance reports by race and ethnicity were not run just at a macro level across all of Kaiser Permanente. It's hard to improve site-specific care when you only have national care data. The data drill-downs for comparative performance were very local. Performance improvement reporting for those operational purposes is very local because care delivery is always very local. Because care is local, the Kaiser Permanente database currently looks at each of those performance levels by region and by care site. That data review discovered that the performance levels and the gaps among the groups varied from site to site. There was a remarkable, overall consistency in intergroup differences across all care sites -- with the care gaps in Honolulu looking very much like the care gaps in Washington, D.C., and that performance tended to look a lot like the care gaps in Sacramento. That was another major learning insight. The performance patterns among the groups looked very similar in all sites. And it was clear, therefore, that shared solutions and joint strategies might be possible to help a diverse set of care sites resolve similar sets of problems.

A HEALTH CARE DISPARITIES SUMMIT WAS CONVENED

The leadership care teams at Kaiser Permanente looked at those gaps and convened an internal care disparities summit to address those issues. The caregivers at the care disparities summit looked at the data and then set up an internal goal of narrowing the performance differences among groups -- with care improvement targets set annually -- with the overall goal of having those intergroup gaps disappear entirely over a couple of years.

That work was done at a very practical and nonacademic level -- because Kaiser Permanente is inherently a care delivery infrastructure and not a policy research organization or an academic think tank.

Before looking at the various steps that were taken inside of Kaiser Permanente to achieve those gap-reduction goals, it is useful to look at the couple of other performance areas where similar care difference gaps were uncovered by the reporting system.

One other point should be made about the blood pressure control chart (Chart 2.2). It is worth mentioning that the average scores for blood pressure control for all patients across all care sites in the rest of the country -- in or out of health plans -- now runs very close to 50 percent of all patients in America who now have their blood pressure under control.[100] Kaiser Permanente had overall performance numbers for blood pressure control that were somewhat closer to those fairly low national care performance levels a decade ago or so. Programs were put in place at that time to improve that area of performance. Those programs succeeded. Kaiser Permanente's overall blood pressure control across the entire care system and across all care teams now averages over 80 percent for all members.[101] Kaiser Permanente currently uses a combination of direct care, medical best practices, patient-focused team care, and systems-supported care to make care better in a continuously improving consistent way for blood pressure control and for multiple other areas of care delivery. The reasons why those approaches are used at Kaiser Permanente are discussed in Chapter Four of this book.

At Kaiser Permanente, the preferred approach of using patient-targeted care that is supported by electronic care tools to help improve care performance in key areas clearly is obviously working for the overall blood pressure control agenda. Lives are being saved. The stroke death rate at Kaiser Permanente has actually dropped by almost 40 percent over the past four years.[102] That particular performance area has been both a high priority and an operational success for Kaiser Permanente, but -- as the data on these charts show -- there were still differences among those racial and ethnic groups inside Kaiser Permanente and -- very specifically -- there is still an intergroup internal performance gap on blood pressure control that needs to be eliminated.

BETA BLOCKER PERSISTENT USE WAS A GAP AREA

Another area where Kaiser Permanente discovered that there were surprising and unsatisfactory differences among ethnic and racial groups was in the persistent use of beta-blockers after a heart attack. Like stroke prevention, preventing both the first and second heart attacks has also been a major performance goal for Kaiser Permanente for a number of years. The overall number of heart attacks is down at Kaiser Permanente by more than 30 percent over the last half decade.[103] Reducing those heart attacks has been an explicit goal of the overall care agenda -- and the appropriate use of beta blockers is a key tool in that effort.

The chart below shows both the overall success levels and the difference in persistence levels by group.

CHART – 2.3

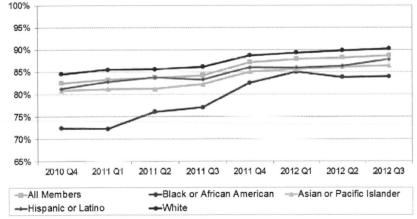

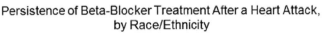

Statistically Significant Differences Exist Between the Highest & Lowest Rates

Persistence of Beta-Blocker Treatment After a Heart Attack, by Race/Ethnicity

© 2012 Kaiser Foundation Health Plan, Inc.

As you can see, the African American success levels for beta blocker use were significantly below the white levels when the measurement process started. That variation and that intergroup performance gap triggered an array of strategies that included focusing on culturally competent training materials, building targeted communications approaches, and improving caregiver coaching skills. Those efforts to deliver better care have resulted in care improvements for all patients on that measure. That very specific, focused improvement plan for minority patients have resulted in a narrowing of the gap among the groups over the past couple of years.

In each area where a performance gap exists, the diversity-focused care strategists at Kaiser Permanente work systematically to figure out best ways of improving the performance levels for the lower scoring patient groups in each gap area. The final chapter of this book includes some segments of the agenda and the care topics that were addressed at the most recent Kaiser Permanente Diversity Conference. A look at those agenda topics can give the reader a sense of the topics being addressed and of the plans that are being used to achieve the various gap-reduction goals. The summit presentations are just a portion of the work being done -- but they are a very important piece of that complete body of work.

CHILDHOOD IMMUNIZATION HAS A STUBBORN GAP

Childhood immunization is another area where there are significant differences in care success levels by race and ethnicity. The set of results that are shown on the charts below follows a slightly different pattern than most other performance levels for the highest and lowest groups compared to many of the other gap areas. This particular chart points out why it is important to understand each gap area issue on its own merits and in its own context.

CHART – 2.4

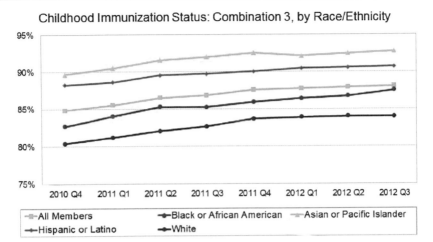

Statistically Significant Differences Exist Between the Highest & Lowest Rates

Childhood Immunization Status: Combination 3, by Race/Ethnicity

Legend:
- All Members
- Black or African American
- Asian or Pacific Islander
- Hispanic or Latino
- White

© 2012 Kaiser Foundation Health Plan, Inc.

In this set of measurements, the highest performing group is clearly the Asian patient population. The immunization rates for those children are among the very best in the world. The Hispanic success levels for childhood immunization are close behind.

The lowest performance levels on this particular quality score are for the white children. Immunizations levels for the white population have been running well below the rates of the other groups inside Kaiser Permanente. That seems to be true in the world outside Kaiser Permanente, as well. That particular difference in vaccination levels by group is triggered largely by an unfortunate array of parental concerns about vaccine safety that seem to be believed most strongly by white patients.[104] Those concerns about various issues of vaccine safety for children have not been supported by actual specific research data. Major studies have shown, in fact, that the suspected and feared link between childhood vaccinations and childhood autism actually does not exist.[105] Some of the early invalidated data that once seemed to show parents that kind of relationship existed turned out not to be accurate data. Kaiser Permanente actually functionally did some of the subsequent scientifically valid autism and vaccination research studies to show that there actually was no link with autism. In spite of those reassuring studies showing that no linkage existed, however, there is still a significant level of concern about that issue with some parents, and that has created a reluctance to have some immunizations done.

As you can see from those group-specific scores, the fear that resulted from the earlier beliefs about that particular set of concerns seems to be most difficult to address for the white patients. There clearly is not a total boycott of immunizations by white parents. Most white parents obviously do immunize their children -- but as you can see on this chart, an unfortunate number do not. This is another area of targeted activity for Kaiser Permanente care teams. Work is underway to create more persuasive materials and better information support that can be used to help those parents deal with those issues for that particular population.

CANCER SCREENING GAPS NEED TO BE REDUCED

One of the most important areas where gaps exist among the population groups is in cancer screening. Studies have shown major screening gaps exist in care sites outside of the Kaiser Permanente care system. The recent national care disparities report highlighted some of the gaps by race and ethnicity. That is important information. Lives are literally at stake. Cancer screening levels can obviously have a huge impact on people's lives. Cancers that are detected early have a much higher cure rate than cancers that are detected late...so early detection clearly saves lives. When people from any ethnic group or race are less likely to have early screening for any cancer -- the people from those groups are much more likely to experience early death. People often underestimate how significant the differences in the death rates can be. It's good to look at real numbers to get a sense of the differences in risk levels.

As the real numbers on the actual cancer survival charts below show, the very lowest survival rates -- and the highest death rates -- for each cancer are for the patients who have their cancer detected very late in the process. The very best survival rates are for the people whose cancers are detected early. When Kaiser Permanente started measuring cancer detection rates by race and ethnicity, some of the same kinds of care gaps among groups that exist for other care performance areas (like blood pressure and beta blocker follow-up) were evident immediately.

The next chart shows the performance levels by group for colon cancer in one of the Kaiser Permanente region -- Southern California. The pattern is basically the same for each of the other regions but the Southern California care team led the way in working to eliminate deaths from this cancer, so their charts are included in this book.

CHART – 2.5

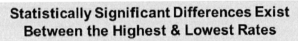

Statistically Significant Differences Exist
Between the Highest & Lowest Rates

Colorectal Cancer Screening, by Race/Ethnicity
Kaiser Permanente Programwide

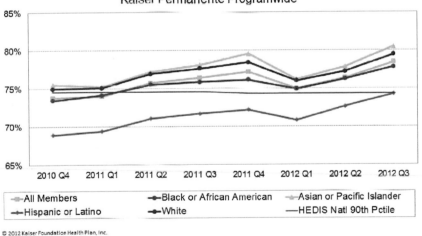

© 2012 Kaiser Foundation Health Plan, Inc.

In each of the Kaiser Permanente regions across the country, the best and highest level of colorectal screening has been for the Asian patients. The lowest screening level for that same cancer in each care site and each geographical site has been for the Hispanic patients.

In this chart, the performance level for colon cancer screening for the Hispanic patients started ten full points lower than the Asian patients. The Hispanic performance levels have now improved significantly but, interestingly, the gap between the groups hasn't narrowed much in four years because the performance levels for all of the other groups have also gone up significantly. The Hispanic screening level inside Kaiser Permanente is now over the 90th percentile for all patients for all other health systems in America who measure that performance, but it is still ten points lower than the best ethnic group level screening levels -- the levels for Asian patients -- inside Kaiser Permanente.

The caregivers involved in reducing that specific gap have learned that there are some relevant differences in attitude, beliefs, and behaviors about cancer screening for many of the Hispanic patients. Those differences needed to be addressed skillfully and with great cultural competence by the care team in order to improve the screening levels for the Hispanic group of patients -- with the ultimate goal of bringing the gap among the groups down to zero.

This is very good work to do.

Colon cancer is a disease where early detection is incredibly important. The next chart shows the actual five-year survival rates for the patients at Kaiser Permanente who have that particular cancer. It's easy to see from the survival rates why early detection of that cancer is so important. On that chart, the survival data for each set of patients is based on how early in the progression of the cancer that the cancer was detected. To offer an interesting comparison data set, that chart also includes the survival rates for similar patients with that same cancer who are being treated in the other cancer programs who also report their performance levels for cancer treatments through the National Cancer Institute's Surveillance, Epidemiology and End Results (SEER) cancer survival database.[106] The SEER sites use that data reporting mechanism as a care improvement tool. It can be extremely useful information for any cancer care site.

CHART – 2.6   **FOR ILLUSTRATIVE PURPOSES ONLY**

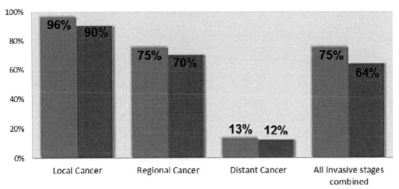

Colorectal Cancer: 5-Year Relative Survival
All Ages, Invasive Cases

■ KP SCAL Patients   ■ SEER Care Site Patients

Stage	KP SCAL	SEER
Local Cancer	96%	90%
Regional Cancer	75%	70%
Distant Cancer	13%	12%
All invasive stages combined	75%	64%

US-SEER Sourced from SEER Cancer Statistics Review, 1975-2009 (Vintage 2009 populations), for invasive cases diagnosed 2002-2008. National Cancer Institute, Bethesda, MD, http://seer.cancer.gov/csr/1975_2009_pops09/, based on November 2011 SEER data submission, posted to the SEER web site, April 2012.

© 2012 Kaiser Foundation Health Plan, Inc.

As you can see, regardless of the care site -- Kaiser Permanente or SEER site -- when the cancer is detected as a local stage-one cancer -- the very earliest stage -- people live longer. More than 96 percent of the patients at Kaiser Permanente and more than 90 percent of the patients being treated at other SEER cancer care sites are still alive five years later when that particular cancer is detected early.

But when that same particular cancer is detected in the late and most widely dispersed stage -- the most dangerous stage -- only 13 percent of the patients at Kaiser Permanente and only 12 percent of the patients at the other SEER cancer care sites are still alive 5 years later. Four percent and eighty-eight percent are a huge difference in the death rate. At Kaiser Permanente only 1 in 20 patients die in that timeframe when that cancer is detected early, and nearly 9 out of 10 patients dies within 4 years when that same cancer is detected late. Early is clearly better.

This survival chart shows the results of the Kaiser Permanente Cancer Program in Southern California. The data for other Kaiser

Permanente care teams is very similar to the Southern California numbers. As noted above, the second bar on the chart shows the results for patients who are being treated in other care sites that report SEER data. Those care sites show a very similar difference in the death rates for patients whose cancers are detected early and patients whose cancers are detected late. That data from all sites clearly confirms and reinforces the Kaiser Permanente belief about the great value of early cancer detection for all patients. The SEER data is for other care systems outside of Kaiser Permanente who are in the National SEER cancer reporting network. SEER sites all use that data for care improvement.

As noted earlier, SEER is an excellent and well-designed cancer reporting mechanism. It helps care systems across the country track their own cancer treatment success levels and also helps those sites compare their own success with other care sites and other care teams.

The cancer centers who report data to the SEER program include many of the best cancer programs in the country. Individual survival rates for other specific cancer programs are not available from SEER by the name of each cancer treatment care site. Each care site only knows their own data and the range of data for other care sites. So the cancer survival charts in this book simply show the average performance of all other SEER sites compared to Kaiser Permanente performance levels for those cancers. People who are seeking care at those other care sites may want to ask those care teams and care sites for their own SEER data.

Overall, for all cases of colorectal cancer, the average five-year survival for all patients who have that cancer at Kaiser Permanente -- regardless of the time of diagnosis -- is 75 percent.[107] The average overall five-year survival rate for all patients with that cancer at the other SEER reporting systems is 64 percent.[108] That significant difference in the survival rates for all stages of that particular cancer is due in large part to the very solid and consistent effort that is being made at Kaiser Permanente to detect that cancer as early as possible for all patients. Early detection is a good priority to have. As those charts show, that is the right thing to do. Early detection clearly saves lives. All other cancer care sites in the world would save more lives if they could also figure out how to detect more of those cancers early.

It is possible that the new accountable care organizations described in Chapter Three may have that agenda and share that early detection priority. The value of that priority is clear.

In any case, the clear difference between the 12 percent survival rate for late detected cancers inside Kaiser Permanente and the 96 percent survival rate for early detected cancers inside Kaiser Permanente shows why Kaiser Permanente places a very high priority in eliminating the performance gap among groups that now exist by race and ethnicity inside Kaiser Permanente relative to early detection of that cancer.

The higher overall cancer survival rates for several key cancers at Kaiser Permanente are driven partly by the strong and often successful focus on early detection processes at Kaiser Permanente. It also explains why disparities in cancer screening levels actually do create disparities in cancer death rates among groups of patients. As noted earlier, the average survival rates go up for all cancers when the cancers are detected early.

It's important to note that the early detection levels only account for part of the overall Kaiser Permanente survival success level, however. When you directly compare survival rates for the late-stage cancers detected at Kaiser Permanente compared to the survival rates for those same late-stage cancers at other care sites across the SEER database, the survival rate for late-stage cancers also tends to still be a bit better for several cancers at Kaiser Permanente, as the next chart shows.

The higher average survival rates at Kaiser Permanente for the cancers that are detected late compared to the average survival levels in the SEER sites for late-stage cancers is due in part to the fact that the care teams at Kaiser Permanente who are treating late-stage cancers are supported by some of the most current care protocols in the world and by one of the best systematic process guidance and support approaches in health care. Those higher success levels for that cancer care are also due in part to the patient-focused team care approach that works to consistently and systematically and continuously improve patient outcomes for various medical conditions for Kaiser Permanente patients.

Colon cancer isn't alone in showing those positive survival rate performance levels. Breast cancer survival rates at Kaiser Permanente also tend to be better overall than the national average. Again -- like the colon cancer data -- that higher survival rate is due in part to early detection -- and it is also due to the slightly better than the SEER average survival rate for the late-stage breast cancers that are detected at Kaiser Permanente.

CHART – 2.7   FOR ILLUSTRATIVE PURPOSES ONLY

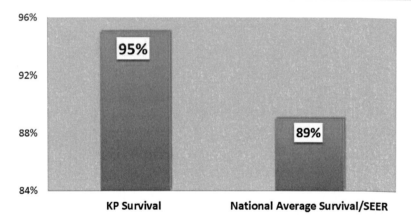

**Breast Cancer: 5-Year Relative Survival
All Ages, Invasive Cases**

US-SEER Sourced from SEER Cancer Statistics Review, 1975-2009 (Vintage 2009 populations), for invasive cases diagnosed 2002-2008. National Cancer Institute, Bethesda, MD, http://seer.cancer.gov/csr/1975_2009_pops09/, based on November 2011 SEER data submission, posted to the SEER web site, April 2012.

© 2012 Kaiser Foundation Health Plan, Inc.

The five-year survival rates for all breast cancer cases at Kaiser Permanente run 95 percent.[109] That compares to the national SEER average survival rate for all breast cancer cases of 89 percent.[110] The late-stage breast cancer five-year survival rates at Kaiser Permanente run at 29 percent[111] -- compared to a SEER average for those late-stage breast cancer patients of 24 percent.[112] The survival patterns based on the stage of diagnosis are exactly the same for all care teams. In all instances -- inside Kaiser Permanente or at any of the other cancer care sites -- cancers that are detected early arc much more likely to be cured. Mammography helps to detect breast cancer early. Kaiser Permanente usually leads the nation on mammography levels. But even though it is true, there are some differences inside Kaiser Permanente by race and ethnicity on that mammography performance area. Those differences in mammography rates by race and ethnicity are also targeted to be eliminated.

CHART – 2.8

FOR ILLUSTRATIVE PURPOSES ONLY

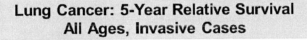

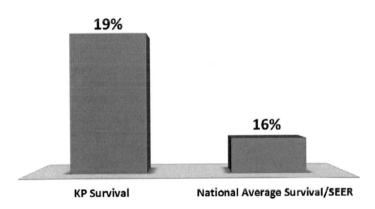

**Lung Cancer: 5-Year Relative Survival
All Ages, Invasive Cases**

19%

16%

KP Survival   National Average Survival/SEER

US-SEER Sourced from SEER Cancer Statistics Review, 1975-2009 (Vintage 2009 populations), for invasive cases diagnosed 2002-2008. National Cancer Institute, Bethesda, MD, http://seer cancer.gov/csr/1975_2009_pops09/, based on November 2011 SEER data submission, posted to the SEER web site, April 2012.

© 2012 Kaiser Foundation Health Plan, Inc.

The chart above shows five-year survival rates for all lung cancer patients. The five-year survival rate for lung cancer patients obviously isn't good anywhere -- regardless of the point of detection. Those grim numbers in lung cancer survival rates for all of the care treatment programs show us all why helping people to stop smoking is so important to do. Relative to care outcomes and care disparities, the higher smoking levels for our minority populations is clearly another key area where persuading people to change behaviors can save lives, and it can help reduce the difference in the life expectancy among groups.

In any case -- for the purposes of this book -- the fact that early detection means higher survival rates for each of the major cancers means that eliminating any care gaps that exist for cancer screening for colon cancer or breast cancer or any other cancer is a very good thing to do. Very specifically, improving the screening levels for Hispanic patients can help eliminate a significant intergroup difference in care outcomes for Hispanic patients -- a gap that doesn't need to exist if the care team works in an organized way to eliminate it. The fact that the gap between the Hispanic patients and the Asian patients still exists at Kaiser Permanente would be obviously more disconcerting if the performance for the best group wasn't also improving so significantly.

HIV CARE OUTCOMES VARY BY RACE IN MOST CARE SITES

One of the most significant areas of care delivery where eliminating differences, disparities and care gaps by race and ethnicity is very important to do relates to HIV care. Like cancer, HIV/AIDS can kill people. For a very long time, the death rate for Black HIV and Hispanic HIV patients in most care settings has been nearly 50 percent higher than the death rate for white patients.[113] That fact was mentioned in the IOM report on care disparities. That historic difference in disease levels and disease outcomes for HIV/AIDS patients was an intergroup care results and care disparity issue that Kaiser Permanente explicitly addressed. Doing well in HIV care was particularly relevant for the Kaiser Permanente care system because Kaiser Permanente has one of the largest populations of HIV patients in the U.S. Kaiser Permanente probably cares for more HIV patients in this country than any other care team -- outside of the U.S. Department of Veterans Affairs (The VA).[114]

The decision was made a number of years ago at Kaiser Permanente to deliver the very best care to the entire HIV population and to deliver that best care for all patients with no disparities in care outcomes among the ethnic and racial groups.

ELIMINATING DISPARITIES IS NOT THE SAME AS ELIMINATING DIFFERENCES

Eliminating disparities in care outcomes is not the same as saying there are no differences in care delivery. Sometimes culturally competent differences in care approaches and care support are actually needed to eliminate an existing gap in care outcomes. The Kaiser Permanente HIV team has built an HIV treatment agenda around each patient -- focusing on individual coaching, teaching, counseling, and treating each patient with the right level of care and with culturally competent information flows and feedback processes.

Focusing on each patient as an individual is the key. Respecting and dealing with cultural variations is a key part of the preferred individual patient focus and process. Getting each individual patient the care plan they individually need is another key element for HIV care success. So how well is that approach of individual focus for each HIV patient going at Kaiser Permanente?

THE VARIATIONS IN HIV DEATH RATES ARE GONE AT KAISER PERMANENTE

This is another area where Kaiser Permanente care performance can be used as a microcosm and template for the entire country. There are a growing number of HIV cases in the country. The average death rates for HIV/AIDS patients tend to vary significantly by race across the total American care system. The outcome of the care for those HIV cases generally varies significantly from group to group and site to site. Kaiser Permanente has now successfully and completely eliminated those outcome differences by race -- proving it actually can be done. The Kaiser Permanente care plans and care support teams have managed to fully achieve their goal of eliminating outcome disparities for that particular category of care. The outcome gap between Black patients and white patients for HIV care is gone. The gap was eliminated by use of patient-specific care plans and by delivering culturally competent care for each patient. Care was improved for all patients, and the care gaps were eliminated in the process.

The overall HIV care that is delivered today by Kaiser Permanente for all of those very diverse patients might well be the best in the world. The disparities in care outcomes have been eliminated, and the overall HIV death rate for all patients at Kaiser Permanente is now less than half of the national average.[115]

So eliminating disparities in outcomes can be done. That HIV/AIDS work shows that it is possible to deliver great care with no significant differences among ethnic and racial groups for a very important category of care.

THE TOOL KIT INCLUDES TEACHING, BEST PRACTICES, AND CULTURAL COMPETENCY

The tool kit that is needed to create consistently great care for all groups of people includes teaching, health literacy for patients, cultural competence for caregivers, language skills, building patient and physician trust, consistent and skillful use of evidence-based clinical guidelines, and targeted patient outreach. Another book needs to be written by Kaiser Permanente that can describe all of those approaches in more detail. The care teams focused on those areas of care have done very creative work aimed at meeting the needs of each set of patients effectively.

The care team approach involves helping patient decision-making, creating outreach when needed to the home settings, and putting in place appropriate levels of community engagement and involvement.

The patients need trusted caregivers, trusted care processes, and trusted sources of information -- with targeted feedback to help each patient stay on the right path. Those are all possible to do -- and continuous improvement processes are supported and enhanced when the care database tracks both care performance and care delivery by patient in a way that reflects and respects the patient's race and ethnicity.

All of those care support tools and core improvement processes and components have been put in place at Kaiser Permanente for multiple areas of care. The processes are being developed and designed. They are far from perfect -- but they tend to be good, workable, and continuously improving processes. The proof of that systematic approach to continuously improving care processes is in creating overall outcome levels for care that are significantly better than the overall outcomes for the country, at large. Lower HIV death rates, higher cancer survival rates, and lower stroke and heart attack death rates at Kaiser Permanente all result from having both best medical practices and systematically supported care delivery in the context of patient-focused, continuously-improving team care.

WHAT NEEDS TO BE IN PLACE TO ACHIEVE THOSE SUCCESS LEVELS ELSEWHERE?

So how did all of that continuously improving care happen?

What kinds of circumstances, situations and business realities were necessary to make that whole care improvement and disparity-reduction agenda possible at Kaiser Permanente? How did Kaiser Permanente end up with consistently improving care results across racial and ethnical groups in important areas of care that are significantly better than the care delivered and received by most people in the rest of the country?

That question is worth asking and answering. It is particularly good to ask and answer that question at this point in our history because trying to solve the issues of care disparities and the widening gaps in care across the entire country without putting some of the key pieces in place that have worked to deliver continuously improving care at Kaiser Permanente are probably doomed to failure in most other care settings. The successes at Kaiser Permanente have not been accidental. The components of the current levels of success for the caregivers need to be understood -- with the goal of taking advantage of the best elements of that agenda and applying it to other settings where care is delivered.

Chapter Four more specifically deals with the issues of what makes Kaiser Permanente able to achieve those goals of reducing care gaps and achieving highest levels of success on care performance while the care gaps are growing in several ways for the rest of the country. Before looking specifically at how Kaiser Permanente has managed to achieve some of those successes, it makes sense to look briefly at how health care financing approaches and care delivery approaches are changing for the overall health care infrastructure of America.

This is a time of change for American health care. We are seeing changes in both care delivery and care financing. The changes are significant. Times of change create real opportunities for improvement. We need to take advantage of the current set of opportunities to achieve the best levels of improvement in the overall delivery of care and to significantly reduce the current set of care disparities and gaps in care.

To do that well, we need to know what those basic opportunities are. That is the next chapter of this book.

CHAPTER THREE

═══════════════════

HEALTH CARE AND HEALTH COVERAGE IS CHANGING

Health care in America today is clearly on the cusp of change. Care delivery is changing significantly in a number of key areas. We are seeing change in both the way we buy care and the way we deliver care. In any time of major change, we can be best served as a nation if we clearly understand the changes that are happening, and then work to figure out what levels and categories of change will be most likely to give us the great outcomes we want to have.

That need to understand the change we want to achieve is particularly true for the area of health care disparities and health care differences. If we want to close the care gaps outlined in the 2012 Health Care Quality Report, we need to support change that will help close those gaps. Change is -- at this point in time -- inevitable. Change is not optional. It will absolutely happen. Both care delivery and care financing are changing, and both will be changing in multiple ways. We need to take advantage of those changes in order to reduce or eliminate the intergroup gaps we have today for key areas of care.

A major change that we know will happen in health care financing can be directly useful as we work to reduce disparities in care. Some of the care disparities exist today because we currently have massive disparities by race and ethnicity relative to who has health insurance coverage.

Today more than 75 percent of the uninsured people in major states such as California come from minority populations.[116] We have major gaps in the percentage of people with health insurance in our minority populations. That current insurance disparity will be at least partially mitigated next year by the new Medicaid program expansion and by the new insurance exchanges that will be created by the Affordable Care Act. The new insurance exchanges will soon be selling subsidized health insurance coverage to low income Americans.

The combination of expanding Medicaid programs and creating subsidized health insurance coverage for low income Americans can only have a positive impact on reducing the current disparity in coverage levels.

The new insurance exchanges that will begin operation on January 1, 2014, will also give all Americans, for the first time since the invention of health insurance, a chance to personally buy individual health insurance, regardless of the health status of the person who is buying the insurance. To take full advantage of that opportunity, we will need to make those new health care exchanges minority-friendly -- with education and promotional campaigns and programs set up to encourage high levels of participation in the exchanges from our minority populations.

That new law will clearly create a very different market for individual insurance. That is one of the inevitable changes mentioned at the beginning of this chapter. It will create a new reality for individual health insurance purchasing. Everyone can now buy coverage. The nature of the coverage that will be sold is also now being defined and modified. Minimum benefit sets have now been set by law -- so the leanest and sparsest insurance plans with the biggest deductibles and the lowest levels of coverage that used to be sold fairly often to individual purchasers will no longer be legal to sell to anyone in the new exchanges.

For people who bought those old, very high deductible plans, premium levels will go up a bit to reflect the new, higher benefit levels.

A newly defined set of preventive benefits will also now be mandated for anyone who buys individual coverage. The prevention part of the new benefit package is fairly robust. That level of prevention services has not been included in most of the high deductible, individual insurance packages that have been sold heavily in recent years in the individual market. So change is happening in care financing. Insurance is changing, benefits are being defined, and access to insurance is now an open door for anyone, regardless of health status.

Those changes should both help reduce disparities in coverage and provide better benefits that can help people with care needs have those needs met, regardless of race or ethnicity.

CARE DELIVERY INFRASTRUCTURE CHANGES ARE HAPPENING, AS WELL

At the same time that the pure health insurance market is changing for several key aspects of coverage, the care delivery infrastructure is also being reorganized, and some elements of the business model we use today to buy care will also now change in some key ways. Those changes in care delivery will also be highly relevant to this book's agenda of ending disparities in care delivery. The changes are badly needed. We have finally begun to recognize the fact at very senior leadership levels in this country that health care delivery in this country has generally been fragmented, splintered, uncoordinated, and too often perversely compensated. We now understand with some clarity at very senior levels of leadership in this country that 75 percent of the care costs in the country are coming from patients with chronic conditions, and 80 percent of the care costs for those patients are coming from the chronic care patients who have multiple care conditions.[117] "Co-morbidities" are the rule, rather than the exception, when we look at the specific patients who generate most health care expenses for our country today. Our leaders are beginning to recognize the fact that those patients who use most of our health care dollars are generally being cared for by an unconnected array of doctors who usually cannot and do not share patient data or coordinate care in any effective way with one another.

Siloed care is a difficult, dysfunctional, often ineffective, and sometimes dangerous way to deliver care. Doctors in this country tend to function in operational silos. Care suffers for far too many people in far too many settings as a result of a massive set of care coordination and care linkage failures. Many patients in this country can tell their own personal stories and their own experiences of extremely debilitating logistical frustration that arises far too often from not having caregivers who can even communicate with one another at the most basic levels.

COORDINATION GAPS CREATE LOGISTICAL BARRIERS FOR PATIENTS

The caregiver communication gaps that exist today among the caregivers in this country can create major inconveniences and significant logistical barriers for far too many patients. Those same exact gaps can also create significant care shortcomings and major logistical dysfunctions for our caregivers.[118]

The caregivers do not intentionally create those connectivity shortcomings.

Our caregivers would almost all strongly prefer to be fully informed about the care being delivered to each of their own patients. Medical care is an information-based science. Doctors can generally provide better care when they have more information about their patients. Far too often, however, we can't create the information flow that is needed to give caregivers that information. As noted above, nearly 80 percent of those care costs for patients with chronic conditions come from people who have comorbidities[119] -- multiple health conditions -- and we have no good way in most care settings to help the doctors get the full set of care information they need for each patient's best care. America needs much better data tools for our caregivers.

That is another key area where care delivery should and will change for the better, if we continue down the key paths we are beginning to put in place. Anyone who delivers care and looks at both the patient's care needs and the logistical challenges in today's approach can figure out some of the key work that needs to be done.

PATIENT-CENTERED MEDICAL HOMES CAN HELP DELIVER TEAM CARE

America obviously needs team care. Patients with multiple health conditions very much need team care. Minority patients who far too often today do not have ongoing relationships with care sites or with specific caregivers very much need team care. We need consistent, science-based, patient-focused team care if we are going to both improve care and reduce the care gaps that exist today for patients in too many care settings.

The need for team care is finally being recognized both by the people who deliver care and by the people who pay for care. Care is changing as a result of that recognition. In many settings, caregivers are now organizing into new care teams. Those new care teams are increasingly being financially and logistically supported by the health plans and by the government agencies that pay for care.

One of the most popular of the new care team arrangements is called the "patient-centered medical home." Tens of thousands of primary caregivers are developing "medical home" skill sets and building the care delivery resources and tool kits that will allow them to deliver team care.[120] The new medical homes are not facilities or actual physical care locations. They are basically "virtual" homes. They are care teams -- not care sites. The new "patient-centered medical homes" are a functional and practical way of organizing the care of patients around care teams. The medical home care teams are usually anchored by one or more primary care physicians, and those doctors tend to be supported in a team setting by nurses and other caregivers. Coordinated care is definitely a better care delivery approach for many patients. Patients who get their care from well-run and well-supported medical homes tend to have significantly fewer care coordination problems and fewer care crises. They spend less time in emergency rooms and spend fewer days in hospital beds.

Those medical-home supported patients usually face fewer of the logistical barriers and the functional screw-ups that can result when all care comes from solo care sites and where each piece of care is delivered by unconnected and unlinked caregivers.[121]

For minority patients -- who are significantly more likely than white patients not to have ongoing relationships with primary care caregivers -- the new medical homes can fill a major care gap and can help reduce some key disparity levels that exist today in care access. Some Medicaid programs in a couple of states that have worked with initial generations and versions of medical homes have seen significant care improvements for their patients and some cost savings as a result of the improved care delivered to their Medicaid enrollees by those homes.

As noted above, both emergency room use levels and the number of needed inpatient hospital days tend to go down -- often significantly -- when patients receive their primary care support from a well-coordinated medical home.[122] More than 10,000 care sites have now met the connectivity and care support standards to be officially and formally certified as medical homes, and almost as many care sites are building their own noncertified medical home capabilities.[123] So that particular change in care delivery is, in fact, happening. The medical homes are a new resource that is changing care for the better -- and we need to understand how to use that new tool kit well to significantly reduce or mitigate intergroup care disparities that exist today for too many people.

The new medical homes are not the only major change in the care delivery business model that is taking place today -- supported by both government programs and private market purchasers. We are also seeing a very important migration of caregivers in many settings to a new "ACO" approach to care delivery. That organizational approach is intended to do an even more effective job in providing patient-focused team care to populations of patients than the medical homes.

ACCOUNTABLE CARE ORGANIZATIONS ARE INTENDED TO CREATE ACCOUNTABLE CARE

A growing number of care sites are currently organizing into what are generally called, "Accountable Care Organizations" -- or ACOs. ACOs also have team care as a key part of their agenda. ACOs tend to be larger in both scope and scale than a basic medical home. The medical homes can do great and much needed work, but they tend to focus their efforts on primary care support teams.

ACOs, by contrast, tend generally to include both medical specialists and hospitals in their caregiver mix. On a broader scale, the ACOs tend to set up multispecialty care teams who are connected with each other in various contractual, functional, and operational ways to meet the total care needs of a given population of patients. The caregivers who form ACOs generally set them up to provide multispecialty team care to their patients in a coordinated and functionally- linked way. The ACOs usually create a focus for each team that is built on the total care needs of a defined set of patients.

That represents another significant change in the way we buy care.

Focusing on the total needs of a population of patients is significantly different than the traditional functional business model for care delivery in this country. The traditional payment model for care is exclusively focused on individual pieces of care that are delivered by and through separate and individual care sites that are organized as separate care business units. Those business units each create piecework care delivery functions that are all funded in pieces by the piecework cash flow model we use today to buy care.

Moving away from that piecework model is another major change in care financing that will result in changes in care delivery that can be very good for the patients who receive care in this country today.

ACOs want and need that new cash flow model to survive and thrive. Moving away from the piecework approach of buying care to buying and selling care as a team by the package is generally a major part of the typical ACO agenda, aspirations, strategy, and clear intentions. Moving away from a pure piecework model isn't always easy to do. When it is done successfully, caregivers face a new and very liberating financial reality. Moving to that cash flow model that pays for packages of care really frees up the care teams in the ACOs to design care around patients instead of designing all care pieces and structure exclusively around what is defined as billable procedures by insurance companies and government payers.

THE PIECEWORK MODEL OF BUYING CARE DOESN'T FOCUS ON OVERALL CARE

As noted earlier in this book, most care in this country today is purchased entirely by the piece. The piecework payment model for buying care is simple. A piece of care is provided by a caregiver to a patient, and each piece of care then generates a separate bill that is then paid for that separate piece of care.

Pieces of care are the absolute focus of that business model for care purchasing -- so pieces of care become the functional unit for the care delivery structure and infrastructure.

The reality is that buying care only by the piece is a highly unlinked and very primitive approach both to care delivery and care purchasing.

One of the unintended consequences of that piecework purchasing approach is a massive accountability void.

The caregivers who function in that piecework model do not have any accountability for the overall care of any patient. The focus and the accountability of each caregiver is purely and directly piecework based -- with the cash flow and the care delivery processes of each caregiver based on delivering and billing for each separate piece of care.

In that model, an asthma patient has to find a care site of some kind to get care when an asthma attack happens. In the piecework care model, no caregiver is responsible or accountable for coordinating the overall care needs of the asthma patient or for preventing future asthma crises. No one is accountable and no one is paid to do anything in a proactive way for those patients. Each care site involved in asthma care in the current piecework payment model simply waits for an active asthma flare-up to happen for some patient, and then the care site and caregiver reacts to each flare-up for each individual patient with the situational and specific unconnected pieces of care delivered to each patient that are relevant to the immediate and incidental care needs that are created in the moment of need by each asthma flare-up.

In that model, no one looks at either the overall care needs of a population or at possible process interventions, or at any of the health related needs of any patient population. No one in the piecework payment model is accountable for creating interventions that might reduce future care needs for any set of patients or for any individual patient. No one is "accountable" in that model for anything preventive or systematic. It is, sadly and perversely, an accountability-free system. There is an almost complete lack of accountability for any level of care other than creating reactive pieces of care in that piecework, cash flow model that deal with the incidents of care and the care pieces that are triggered when individual care needs happen for a patient. Major opportunities to do highly effective interventions and preventions for various diseases do not happen very often in that business model because no one in the piecework model is accountable for doing that work and no one is paid for doing that work.

The Piecework Model is Neither Accountable or Organized

That lack of accountability is particularly unfortunate for lower income patients who generally can benefit significantly by having proactive care support that can -- when done well -- eliminate most asthma attacks and also very significantly reduce the complication levels for diabetes, congestive heart failure, and each of the other chronic diseases that are more than 75 percent of the costs of care in this country. [124]

Data shows us that the Hispanic, African American, and Native American patients are all less likely today to have even one primary caregiver, much less a team of accountable caregivers who work on those aspects of care.[125] Disparities and care gaps result from that disparity in access to primary care, team care, and proactive care.

The new ACO approach and the new medical homes are both intended to help solve that longstanding problem of not having any part of the care delivery infrastructure being either systematic or proactive about the actual delivery of care or the future care needs of any patients. By contrast, an asthma patient in a well-run medical home or ACO setting will have an immediate, clearly designated pathway to care when that care is needed. Those asthma patients who are in a medical home setting also generally will also have a designated caregiver in their medical home -- typically a doctor or a nurse -- who will help each patient both avoid future asthma crises and help minimize the damage levels from the crises that do happen.

That is much better care. It is a major change in care delivery.

Building medical homes and accountable care organizations that can perform those functions is obviously very important work. Being proactive is a very different way of delivering care and of thinking about care for most care sites and for the vast majority of patients.

The opportunities created by proactive care are not insignificant. Good studies have shown that up to 75 percent of the major asthma crises that result in hospital stays could be averted or prevented with the right proactive care approaches.[126]

Proactive Care Can Reduce Asthma Attacks and CHF Crises

The new accountable care organizations are being set up to deal with those issues and to take advantage of the opportunities presented by care reengineering. The ACOs are intended to be "Accountable," "Care" centered, and "Organized."

"Accountable" is a very important word and a key part of the ACO concept. "Care" is equally important. The new ACOs will each be "accountable" as a "care" team for the total care needs of a given population of people. The ACOs will -- if the model is done well -- have a positive impact on the total care needs of a given population of people. The multiple levels of highly effective proactive care approaches that are now possible for asthma patients will generally be built into each well-run ACO's operating agendas. Those same proactive approaches and crisis-mitigation strategies will be created for multiple other health conditions, if the ACOs and medical homes have the right business model and the right focus on overall care.

There is a long list of really important opportunities available for effective proactive care.

Congestive Heart Failure Needs Proactive Care Approaches

Congestive heart failure (CHF) is another very good example where patients can achieve significant benefits from proactive care. Very clear proactive team care opportunities obviously exist for most patients with CHF. Like asthma attacks, CHF crises are terrible, painful, sometimes terrifying, generally debilitating, and potentially fatal events. A patient having a CHF crisis is drowning in their own fluids. Most CHF patients are eventually killed by their disease. Dying of CHF can be a very painful death. In the wrong care settings, that death can be preceded by multiple, very painful, and often terrifying CHF crisis events.

That is not a necessary pattern of care.

Roughly half of those debilitating CHF crises can actually be averted or prevented by the right package of proactive care.[127] Proactive team care is far better care for those heart failure patients. That proactive care approach for heart failure patients typically does not happen in very many care settings today because of the standard piecework care delivery business model we use now to buy CHF care. That lack of proactive care for CHF patients is not atypical. As noted earlier, the current piecework business model we use to buy care is very perversely designed for multiple areas of care. In that piecework payment model, a congestive heart failure crisis can create 30,000 to 50,000 dollars in revenue — while preventing the CHF crisis entirely for a patient typically generates no revenue at all. Likewise, heart attacks generate significant caregiver cash flow, where preventing heart attacks generates no financial reward. We have thousands of billing codes for procedures -- and not one billing code for a cure.

That payment approach answers the question of why preventive care doesn't happen in any effective way for far too many patients who really need it.

BUSINESSES DO NOT REENGINEER AGAINST THEIR OWN SELF INTERESTS

Health care is a business. Every care site tends to be a separate business. It isn't a good thing for any business in any industry not to have revenue.

Businesses with no revenue almost always fail. In any industry, businesses that have no revenue simply go bankrupt or just disappear. That need for revenue is just as true of health care businesses as it is true for businesses in every other industry. So when we buy care entirely by the piece, the health care businesses of this country often cannot afford to do any of the efficient things that eliminate any of those pieces, because those efficiency-based changes that eliminate unneeded steps literally generate no revenue for the care site. There is no revenue for most care sites unless a procedure is done for a patient.

As noted earlier, up to 75 percent of the asthma crises that happen today could be averted -- with the right proactive care.[128] Half of the congestive heart failure crises could be averted -- again, with the right proactive care.[129] Nearly half of heart attacks and 40 percent of strokes could be eliminated with the right proactive care.[130] Proactive care is rare in American health care because prevention generates minimal revenue for the piecework care business -- but each of those actual crises that do happen to patients for any of those conditions can generate 10,000 to 40,000 dollars in piecework revenue for those care sites. So we obviously very directly encourage, incent, and reward crises-based care and poor care outcomes when we buy care only by the piece.

MEDICAL HOMES SELL PACKAGES OF CARE -- NOT JUST PIECES OF CARE

The new approaches to care delivery will only work if buyers channel cash to make them happen.

Caregivers need cash. That need to have available cash for a care team to do prevention work for patients is why most of the new patient-centered medical homes are set up with some level of per-patient cash flow that pays each medical home a fixed amount of money for a package of care rather than just paying the care site by the piece for incident-based pieces of care. That's also why the new ACOs that are being formed are working out their own financial arrangements with payers and with the government to create a cash flow that will pay their care teams for packages of care rather than just being paid for pieces of care. That model of being paid by the package can create the needed resources for creative and effective proactive care. So this is an area where change is happening and where change is badly needed. The current financial model clearly needs to evolve. The new ACOs need a cash flow volume and a cash flow stability that will allow them to cut asthma crises and CHF crises and heart attacks and strokes in half for their patients without going bankrupt.

The value for both care quality and care affordability that can result from creating those new business models for care is becoming increasingly obvious.

So -- as noted at the beginning of this chapter -- care is changing. Buyers are beginning to lead the way, because the benefits of some aspects of change are so obvious that they deserve buyer support.

Medicare is now encouraging the creation of both ACOs and patient-centered medical homes. That is a very good strategy for Medicare to follow. Most major health plans in America are attempting to create connected contractual relationships with caregivers that will allow the health plans to have the benefits of both team care and proactive care delivery. A lot of very creative work is going on in various settings across the country for both caregivers and payers to make that all happen. We need to make sure that our minority group populations who have both been disproportionately uninsured and disproportionately underserved by team care will benefit fully from those new care delivery approaches. Ideally, the data reporting that will be required from the new ACOs and medical homes will allow care tracking by race and ethnicity -- very much as it is being done today at Kaiser Permanente. That is a good and functional data model to follow if the goal is to reduce disparities in care.

THE TOOL KITS FOR CARE GET BETTER EVERY DAY

At the same time that the need for proactive team care is becoming obvious to buyers and policymakers, there is a separate and very important revolution going on relative to the new tool kits that can be used to support care delivery. The new systems supported care delivery tool kit can also help reduce or mitigate the care gaps that exist for groups of patients today. For centuries, health care has functioned with a very basic and relatively crude set of information resources. The key information tool used most often by caregivers in this country today is literally ancient. Paper. Paper medical records are the rule. Most care sites still use paper records that are stored at each care site where care is delivered. That dependence on paper surprises a lot of people, but the truth is that most medical information in this country is still maintained on paper medical records. That is not good for any groups of patients.

Paper is an inferior, dysfunctional, and sometimes dangerous data tool for health care. Ideally, doctors who are taking care of a patient should have all of the information about each patient easily available to the caregiver at the exact time when care is delivered. Medicine is, at its core, an information-based science. To have caregivers delivering care with major information gaps in the exam room or having hospitals delivering care with major information gaps for the caregivers about each patient -- and with major gaps also in place for too many caregivers about the best and most important medical science -- the combinations of those factors creates some real problems in the way we deliver care.

WE NEED ELECTRONIC DATA ABOUT PATIENTS

Those problems do not need to exist.

Delivering care with major information gaps is a particularly bad way to deliver care when we already have much better approaches and functional tools that are easily available and that work really well when they are used. Paper is clearly the worst data recollection and storage approach -- other than relying on pure unassisted caregiver or patient memory. Information about patients that is stored on paper medical records tends to be splintered -- because each care site usually has its own pieces of paper with information that is specific and limited to the exact pieces of care that are delivered to each patient at that specific site. The paper records for any given patient at any given care site are almost always incomplete. They are always functionally inert -- unable to link with one another in any way. In some cases and in many settings, the paper records are at least partially illegible. Paper records in any given care site are almost always inaccessible for many elements of patient care. Those paper records at any site are almost always inaccessible to the caregivers at other care sites who serve the same patient.

So our primary source of medical information about patients in this country still tends to be incomplete, sometimes inaccurate, inherently inert, completely inactive, and generally inaccessible segments and slices of data that are stored in inconvenient ways on isolated pieces of paper.

Better tools exist now to do that work. They should be used.

Those extensive data deficiencies should not be acceptable to the patients of America, or to the government programs or the private employers who pay for most medical care in this country through their benefit plans.

DATA DEFICIENCIES MAKE DEALING WITH DISPARITIES MORE DIFFICULT

Those data deficiencies obviously make dealing with health care disparities much more difficult, because it is almost impossible to track, monitor, or report on care performance for any care site when the needed information is locked up in pieces of paper. Those data deficiencies should be particularly unacceptable to us all when we now spend $2.8 trillion in total as a country on care.[131] Our care delivery infrastructure absorbs so much cash every year now that if American health care were a separate national economy, it would be the fifth largest economy in the world.[132]

That is enough money to expect that caregivers should have complete data about each patient and to expect that the information about each patient should be available to each patient's caregiver when that information is needed at the point of care. That is also enough money to expect that there should be rich streams of data available to compare care performance and to track basic patterns of care. Detecting disparities takes data. We need to detect disparities in order to correct them. We should be able to identify care disparities almost as soon as they happen. We can do that if we have the right set of data and the right mechanisms in place to get access to that data.

That specific point about the new tool kit that is needed for care delivery is highly relevant to this book on care delivery disparities because it is almost impossible to detect, measure, track, or improve any disparities in any care sites or any care settings without adequate data about care.

The people who wrote the 2003 IOM Report on care disparities said that data was needed to detect, improve, and reduce disparities.[133] They were entirely correct. It is hard to reduce disparities without data about those disparities -- and paper data is impossible to use as an information resource to support that work.

ELIMINATING DISPARITIES IS IMPOSSIBLE WITHOUT DISPARITIES DATA

Eliminating care gaps is functionally impossible without data reporting systems that let the caregivers in each site and care setting know when disparities exist. That need for data is true in all care sites. Look back at Chapter Two in this book. The Kaiser Permanente caregivers had no clue that any of the care disparities and care gaps that were outlined on the performance charts that were shown in that prior chapter even existed for those patients until each category of care was tracked by group, measured by group, and then compared by the group and by the site to the performance of the other groups and the other care sites.

USING DATA IS IMPOSSIBLE WHEN DATA DOESN'T EXIST

The logic involved is pretty simple and it is very pure. Using data is impossible when data doesn't exist. A major first step in improving care is to have data that allows care to be measured. As this country begins to build our new ACOs and to create our new medical home care teams, we need to build that wisdom and that tool kit into each of those new care sites. They will each need data to make care better, and they will need data to eliminate disparities. We need data to track care and we really need data to deliver the best care to each patient. When care is measured and recorded, care can improve. Having data about each patient available to caregivers at the point of care is extremely important as a key tool needed to deliver the best care to each patient. That piece of information is extremely important for a book on health care disparities and that point about the need for data is more important today than it has ever been.

We are moving to a new world for American health coverage. More people will be insured. That expanded insurance coverage will create a significant set of opportunities for care improvement. When 10 to 15 million more Americans become covered by Medicaid, that expansion of coverage for those very low-income people will massively shrink the health care insurance disparities that exist now for those sets of people.

We need to make sure that the programs that we put in place in each state that expands Medicaid deal directly and explicitly with the issues of needed team care and needed care data.

The truth is, however, that the pure expansion in insurance coverage will not automatically eliminate any actual care delivery disparities for anyone with either Medicaid coverage or private insurance. Eliminating or reducing our insurance disparities is a good thing, but that particular gap reduction doesn't make our care delivery disparities disappear. Lower income people will still be less likely to have available care sites and consistent access to basic care than higher income people. For lower income people to receive the best levels of care, we will need a data flow infrastructure and a care delivery strategy that makes the care data for those newly insured patients both electronic and portable. It is even more important now for newly insured, low income people to have their caregiver teams armed with a workable set of care data -- because care for lower income people tends to be even more splintered by site and by caregiver than care for higher income people.

The good news is that when the care data is both electronic and linked, care can get better. The care infrastructure that functions at Kaiser Permanente is consistently and constantly proving that theory and that contention about the value and the potential for that data to improve care to be true at multiple levels. When easily accessible data exists about care, caregivers can do a better job for each patient and the overall levels of care can become both more consistent and safer.

Data Is Needed to Make Hospitals Safer

Safety is an important issue for American health care. We also need to address patient safety as we address disparities in care.

One area that proves that point about the sheer value and functional benefits of data for the process of improving care relates to hospital safety. We actually have significant problems today in this country in many areas relative to hospital safety. One of the unfortunate aspects of health care in America today is that 1.7 million Americans enter a hospital every year and get an infection they did not have on the day they were admitted to the hospital.[134] Those infections kill people -- and they also cost a lot of money.

Studies have shown that the hospitals that serve the most Black patients tend to have consistently higher death rates -- and those higher death rates are due to the care system -- not the patients.[135]

There are far too many infections in our hospitals today.

We clearly need to make changes in the way we buy care.

We need a business model for purchasing care that does not financially reward the care sites where infections occur. ACOs can make that happen. The new ACO cash flow approaches should be set up so that the ACOs have a strong incentive to create safer care and so the care sites are not penalized financially when care does get safer. Care safety and the need to create systematically safer care are not insignificant issues.

Sepsis -- a blood stream infection -- is actually the number one cause of death in American hospitals.[136] Most people do not know that to be true. More people actually die of sepsis in hospitals than die of cancer, heart disease, or stroke .[137] Twenty percent of seniors who died in California hospitals died of sepsis.[138]

DATA-FREE BELIEFS CAN BE SINCERE AND WRONG

That is a tragedy. An even bigger tragedy is that most of those sepsis deaths could have been prevented. The next chart shows the reduction in sepsis death rates that happened at a dozen California hospitals. That chart also shows why data is so extremely important. Before any measurement of sepsis deaths was done, all of these hospitals believed they were delivering great sepsis care. All of the hospitals had key people in each site who were entirely well-intentioned. All of the care sites on that chart knew the basic science of sepsis care. But the chart shows that the care for sepsis patients was obviously not as effective in each of the hospitals. Some hospitals had a much higher death rate from sepsis. Learning that fact about the difference in the mortality levels was a golden gift to all of the hospitals on that chart because it gave those low-performing hospitals both the context and the perspective they needed to get better at treating sepsis. And -- because care processes were focused on when the data became available -- that same data also ultimately helped the higher performing hospitals get better. Those 12 hospitals -- as you can see from that sepsis mortality chart -- all used that new knowledge about their care results to actually improve care. A lot of lives have been saved in those 12 hospitals over the past couple of years because that data did the extremely important work of helping the low-performing care sites know that they were not delivering care at optimal levels.

Before the data reports were done, every hospital on that chart believed strongly that their sepsis care was the right care. Everyone believed their performance levels were high. That was, however, a data-free belief. Data-free beliefs are not an optimal care management tool. Only real data about real performance can actually create the working context for real performance improvement. Using real-time and accurate data about care processes and care outcomes is particularly true for sepsis.

CHART – 3.1

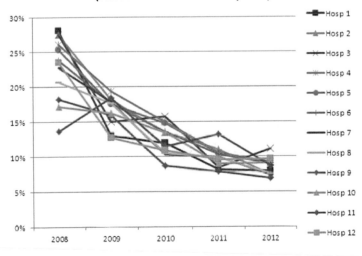

Basic Inpatient Mortality Among Patients with Sepsis
(Kaiser Permanente Hospitals)

© 2012 Kaiser Foundation Health Plan, Inc.

Sepsis Care Lends Itself to Process Improvement

The sepsis care process really lends itself to systematic process design and redesign work by teams of caregivers. There is a "golden hour" for each patient in sepsis care where the death rate can be cut in half with the right care.[139] Hospitals who take a systematic approach to care improvement can functionally learn to do the exact right things in that golden hour -- like, getting each patient's lab tests back to the patient's caregiver in 15 minutes or less rather than letting those lab tests for each patient go through the normal hospital lab test result response cycles and information distribution systems. The normal response cycle for routine hospital lab tests can take one to four hours in many care settings. It's hard to treat your sepsis patient with the right drugs and do that lifesaving treatment for that patient inside that "golden hour" time frame if the lab tests that diagnose the disease for each patient do not come back to the care floor until two hours or four hours or even six hours later.

Many lives are saved in hospitals when the lab tests for sepsis care get back quickly enough to make a bigger difference in each patient's care. So each hospital who wants to reduce their sepsis deaths needs to reengineer their lab processes and information flow to make that targeted result happen.

When that overall sepsis mortality-reduction work is done well, the hospitals not only track sepsis deaths -- they also can put processes in place that measure how many minutes it took to diagnose each patient and how many minutes it took to get the right drugs to each patient. Continuous improvement in care delivery benefits hugely through the skillful use of the right set of critically important process data to support care process improvement.

The hospitals that continuously improve their processes have shown they can cut sepsis deaths by more than half. They can also reduce lifetime patient damage for the survivors of sepsis. That is another key point to understand about the extremely high value and benefit of getting sepsis care right for patients. When the sepsis patient gets the right treatment in the right rapid time frame, the patients who survive their sepsis infection and go home from the hospital also tend to have a lot less permanent or long-term damage than the patients who get their sepsis treatment more slowly -- in two or four or six hours. The patients who get slow care and who still survive to go home from the hospital are significantly more likely to be permanently damaged from sepsis than the patients who get fast care and also survive. Patients in the best care sites are much more likely to go home undamaged rather than ending up in a lifelong care setting -- with permanent support needed to deal with permanently damaged internal organs.

For low income people -- often minority patients being treated in low- performance care sites -- being permanently damaged by sepsis makes an economically challenged financial reality for the patients even worse. Minority patients very much need best sepsis care. Not weak or inadequate sepsis care.

THE NEW ACOS NEED TO DO PROCESS IMPROVEMENT

We need to understand how the care improvement process works. Speed is clearly essential to improve results for some areas of care. Speed doesn't happen spontaneously. It also doesn't happen consistently. Process improvement work is needed to create speed. Data can help deliver, create, and support improvements in care delivery speed. Data also lets us improve care and track care. ACOs need to work hard to design the right data flow. Data is badly needed for the new care delivery world, and the existence of data can be supported in important ways by the new insurance environment we are moving into. The new ACOs should be data-focused at key performance levels. The process-aligned model can work. Suggesting that ACOs build that tool kit isn't a theoretical or hypothetical suggestion. The fact is -- Kaiser Permanente functions now as a kind of ACO -- and the ACO tool kits described above clearly offer functional value in that setting. Kaiser Permanente is currently proving the value of having data-supported care in an accountable care setting to be something that all of the new ACOs should aspire to achieve.

A major key to the success in care improvement and disparity reduction work at Kaiser Permanente is to have all of the patient data on the computer. The problems of paper-based data were described earlier. Paper is no longer used for those purposes in either the Kaiser Permanente hospitals or in the Kaiser Permanente medical offices. All of the data is computerized. That work to computerize all patient records was done for that entire care infrastructure as a full package of interconnected data flows because the paper medical records that were used in the past were functionally inferior, and they resulted in significantly less effective care for Kaiser Permanente patients.

What can the rest of the country learn from that experience?

The primary conclusion that can be learned is that electronic medical records should be the standard way we all record data about care in all care sites in this country. Paper medical records should disappear.

For individual patients, the care teams need computerized care plans. The care team members also need tools that support patient-specific care tracking. As noted earlier, Kaiser Permanente has managed to cut the death rate for HIV patients to half of the national average using those kinds of tools.[140]

Kaiser Permanente also eliminated the racial care disparities in the process for HIV patients by building individual computer-supported care plans that are built around each patient -- then using the entire computerized care data tool kit as a prompt and a support system for follow-up care. The tools that are available when data is computerized are obviously far better than the care support tools that are anchored in a paper database.

NEW CARE TOOLS COULD REVOLUTIONIZE CARE

The next generation of care support tools is going to be even more impressive and more useful than the old care tools. New tools are being developed daily. Some of the new tools are amazing new pieces of technology that track and monitor patients remotely at low costs with a higher degree of accuracy and great convenience.

New remote monitoring tools that exist today can actually do a functional EKG test from a low cost device connected to a smartphone. New technology can track activity levels, blood pressure, and the symptoms of multiple diseases, and do it at remarkable low expense levels.

To get care right and to make care the most affordable in the future for people of all races and ethnicities, we need to embrace that new set of care support tools, and we need to incorporate those tools effectively in a team-based way into the overall way we deliver care -- with an underlying support of electronic medical records for each patient. Team care can be enhanced and enabled with the new connectivity tools. The business model of care needs to support that process. We need the new ACOs and the new medical homes to have a cash flow that enables and encourages them to use and embrace that new set of tools. We need to remove economic and functional barriers to the more effective use of those tools, and we need to link those new tools to team care in increasingly effective ways.

That will not happen unless we choose as a nation to make it happen and unless the primary purchasers of health care create the cash flow that will enable it to happen.

We Need the New Tools to Support Team Care

We could be starting down some dysfunctional paths for some of those new tools in their current iterations.

Too many of those lovely new tools are being set up today without the right linkage capabilities or linkage strategies. That is unfortunate. The new tools will become their own electronic data silos if that level of isolation happens. Creating a new set of isolated electronic data silos that will replace the old set of paper-based, nonfunctional isolated data silos isn't significant progress. Replacing isolated paper silos with new isolated electronic silos would clearly be the wrong path to go down. To eliminate care disparities, we need best care, we need accountable care, we need connected care, and we need care that is supported by the new array of care tools. We very much need the data being made available by those new tools to be universally linked with each other to create optimal care for our patients.

So as we look at the new care tools, the new care organizational models, and at the expanded number of people who will now have coverage instead of being uninsured, this is obviously the time to make some important decisions about key aspects of delivering care and collecting care and sharing care information. We particularly need to make a few important decisions in each of those areas if we want to eliminate the current set of disparities in care delivery and the perverse differences in care outcomes.

THE NEW ACOS NEED TO LEARN FROM SUCCESS

This time of change should be a time of progress and advancement.

It would be a mistake to simply insure millions of additional people and not both improve care delivery and care data flows at the same time. The new accountable care organizations are being created to do some of that care improvement and data flow improvement work. That is the right thing to do. The new ACOs can be well-designed, well-structured, and well-incented. If those care organizations are paid with a cash flow that enables them to sell care by the package and not just sell care by the piece, those new care teams will have a high likelihood of success.

Their likelihood of success will probably be enhanced if they understand and use some of the operational and strategic approaches that have been designed, implemented, and continuously improved. In the Kaiser Permanente care infrastructure over the past several years, it has been involved in an overall continuous improvement process that has anchored very basic accountable care organization functionality for those care teams for a number of years. It is worth understanding that functionality and its component parts at this time of great change in both care delivery and care financing, because the other organizations who want to deliver accountable care can benefit from both the mistakes made and the successes that have been created in that ongoing and large-scale accountable care and team care context.

The next chapter deals with some of those learnings and explains some of the basic guidelines, strategic directions, and functional approaches that have proven to have value for those 9 million patients and their caregivers.

CHAPTER FOUR

LEARNING FROM A LONGSTANDING FOCUS ON ACCOUNTABLE CARE TO IMPROVE CARE FOR EVERYONE

One of the very best ways of reducing care disparities in America is to improve care for everyone. A rising tide of continuously improving, better care will bring care for all groups to a consistently higher level. That actually should be possible to do. It may, in fact, be the only way we can eliminate some disparities that exist today in care delivery. That is true because we can't focus on improving care for just a subset of our population in a functionality vacuum. The same tools that can be used to reduce disparities are the same tools we need to use to improve care for everyone. We need to put the tools and processes in place to improve care for everyone, and then we will have those tools in place to fix disparities and to eliminate the gaps we now have in care delivery and care outcomes.

That work is possible to do. This is very much the right time to do that work. As noted in the prior chapter, the health care policy agenda in this country is increasingly focused on creating various kinds of team care, data-supported care, and accountable care for all Americans. Those areas of focus on improved care functionality will each be very useful in reducing care disparities. Medicare, Medicaid, and private payers are all trying to figure out how to create and support care delivery approaches that will improve overall care by making care both better and more affordable.

As noted earlier -- it costs less to prevent an asthma crisis than it does to treat an asthma crisis. The government-funded portion of that care improvement agenda will be particularly important for the key populations where significant care disparities exist today. Those tools are needed even more for the patients whose care is less than adequate today. The people who are advocates for computer-supported care, patient-focused team care, and the use of process improvement techniques to enhance care delivery tend to believe that care will get better for all patients with the right focus, the right business model, and the right tool kit.

People who look closely at the issues of care disparities that were outlined earlier in this book also tend to share the belief that we need better data-gathering as a nation, and we need better care support tools for all caregivers and for all patients if we want to successfully address and remedy the care disparity issues that exist today, in the most focused and effective ways. The perceived need for those tools is well-founded. Those are the tools we need to do that work. As noted earlier, both of those beliefs and those tools are being tested today in an operational way in the Kaiser Permanente care settings.

The theory that says one of the best ways to reduce care disparities is to make care better for all patients is happening today for the 9 million extremely diverse patients and the even more diverse care teams at Kaiser Permanente. Data shown earlier in this book looks at care improvement at Kaiser Permanente overall and by race and ethnicity. That overall data and that group-specific data should be encouraging for the rest of the country. Those improvements in performance inside the Kaiser Permanente infrastructure of care delivery clearly represent the kind of gap-reduction successes that strong advocates of disparity improvement and gap closures would like to see happen for the whole country.

As noted earlier, this is a particularly good time to learn from that work at Kaiser Permanente because the new medical homes and the new ACOs that are forming in multiple settings all need to create a functional tool kit so that caregivers in those settings can build in several ways on the tool kits that are already in place at Kaiser Permanente.

What can the new ACOs and medical homes learn from those existing Kaiser Permanente tool kits?

KAISER PERMANENTE IS A FUNCTIONING ACO NOW

The first point for those new care organizations to understand is that Kaiser Permanente is functionally an accountable care organization now. Kaiser Permanente is a prototype ACO. Kaiser Permanente sells packages of care now and does not use a piecework payment model today for its cash flow. As noted earlier in this book, other health care businesses in this country almost all bill separately for each piece of care. Kaiser Permanente has a total per-patient cash flow as its business model and actually has no internal bills for any elements of care. Each Kaiser Permanente member today buys a package of care. They buy that package by paying a monthly premium. The monthly premium is a flat amount paid per member, per month. That premium can be paid by the member, by the employer, by the government, or by various combinations of those payers.

The key to understand is that the basic cash flow model for Kaiser Permanente is to sell a full package of care for a monthly price. That cash flow from each member goes to Kaiser Permanente as a monthly payment package, and that money is then functionally used as needed to deliver both the care and the prevention services that Kaiser Permanente members and patients need.

It is true from a cash flow perspective that some patients at Kaiser Permanente have chosen to buy deductible benefit plans. Some people bought those plans from Kaiser Permanente to reduce their premium levels -- and those people with deductible plans do pay individual prices for the pieces of care that are needed after they meet their personal deductible amount. But the economic reality is that the cash flow from those payments for pieces of care from those patients represents a very small portion of the Kaiser Permanente total revenue. Those payments do not change the basic business model for care. Inside Kaiser Permanente, there are hospital budgets, but there are no internal hospital prices.

All of the Permanente doctors receive a salary. Permanente physicians are not paid based on an accumulation of fees that are created by individual pieces of care that each doctor delivers. Fees are not an internal cash flow reality, and fees are not linked to any doctor's individual cash flow at Kaiser Permanente. That means that the Permanente doctors can focus on delivering needed care for patients without being affected financially by any of their care decisions. Salaries are the physician compensation approach. Salaries create a very different care context for caregivers than piecework payment approaches.

The Mayo Clinic, the Cleveland Clinic, and the Geisinger Clinic also all use salaries instead of fees as the way they pay their physicians. Salaries are a very liberating way for caregivers in those care settings to be paid because the take- home pay of any physician can't be adversely affected by doing or not doing unneeded but profitable individual care procedures.

Many of the people who are designing the new ACOs in care sites across the country are working to design cash flow models that move away from piecework payments to package-based purchases of care.

The new ACOs tend to understand the obvious advantages of selling packages of care, and most of the new ACOs are attempting to create cash flow approaches that more closely resemble and parallel the macro cash flow approach that exist at Kaiser Permanente. That is a good direction for those ACOs to follow.

MAKING CARE SAFER AND BETTER BECOMES A GOOD BUSINESS DECISION

That is a very good strategy for those care sites to follow.

Receiving a prepayment amount every month for each patient changes the overall business model of health care organizations. There are a number of significant benefits for health care organizations and care delivery that result from not being paid for care by the piece. Making care better and safer for the patient becomes a wise business decision instead of creating a revenue loss for the caregivers when the care teams can function in a prepaid, package-based care setting.

The Kaiser Permanente Package Payment Hospitals Have -- for Example -- Fewer Hospital-Acquired Pressure Ulcers

Kaiser Permanente hospitals have incredibly low levels of hospital-acquired pressure ulcers, for example.[141] In the rest of the country, on average, 7 to 15 percent of all patients end up with those painful, disfiguring and sometimes fatal ulcers.[142] The number of those unfortunate pressure ulcers tends to be higher in some of the hospitals serving minority patients. The standard business model of care responds in a very perverse way to the cash flow relating to those ulcers. Those hospitals that get paid for all care by the piece generally receive paid additional fees for those patients that are based on the additional care needs that are created by those ulcers. That payment for those damaged patients can create a lot of revenue. On average, more than 7 percent of patients get those ulcers. Some hospitals have over 10 percent of their patients with those ulcers.[143]

In the Kaiser Permanente-owned hospitals, however, where care is sold by the package and not by the piece -- the average level of pressure ulcers is now under 1 percent of all patients.[144] One percent is a very low number. Several Kaiser Permanente hospitals have not had one single stage 2 or higher pressure ulcer for more than a year.[145] That is far better care for those patients.

So the reality is -- for that very common patient-damaging infection -- the very highly diverse caregivers at Kaiser Permanente deliver spectacular, incredibly focused, very highly skilled care for the hugely diverse Kaiser Permanente patient population to keep those ulcers from happening. That level of care success isn't accidental or easy. The care levels and the patient-focused care commitment required by the hospital-based care teams to achieve that high level of care quality are intense. As a result, the success levels for pressure ulcers in those hospitals may be the best in the world. The cash flow for those ulcers that occur at Kaiser Permanente works like a well-designed ACO cash flow should work. There is an increase in care quality and there is no decrease in care revenue at Kaiser Permanente when the number of pressure ulcers has been hugely reduced. In other piecework-reimbursed care settings, that much safer and much better level of care for those patients could actually create a significant revenue loss for the piecework paid care sites.

That is an important example to keep in mind as the country considers expanding the use of both ACOs and medical homes and applying them to programs that serve our minority populations. Safety in those care settings can be enhanced by not financially rewarding the consequences of unsafe care and by actually rewarding the consequences of safe care.

BEING PAID BY THE PIECE HAS SEVERAL NEGATIVE, DYSFUNCTIONAL, AND PERVERSE CONSEQUENCES

Being paid by the piece has a number of very perverse and completely unintended consequences. Care volume is one problem. That is the most widely known problem with piecework payment approaches. Most economists who look at health care issues understand the sheer care volume incentives that inherently result for any vendor for any product when the vendor is being paid entirely by the piece. The fact that we have more CT scans done in this country than any other country in the world other than Japan is obviously based at least in part on the usually highly profitable fees that are paid to each scan owner when each scan is done.

There are many other comparable examples of care volumes and patterns of care that are based more on caregiver revenue opportunities than patient care needs. Cesarean-sections are a good example. C-sections are often pointed to as an area where the volume incentives inherent in a piecework payment model that pays much more money for a C-section compared to the payment for a normal delivery creates perverse, unfortunate, and medically inappropriate care volumes. The relationship between piecework payment incentives and the care unit volume for multiple areas of care is well-understood by most health care economists.

Piecework Payment Cripples Care Improvement

That volume-trigger and incentive is not, however, the biggest economic flaw in that particular payment model. The biggest flaw in the piecework model is the fact that being paid by the piece cripples, penalizes, stifles, and stands as a direct barrier against most care improvement agendas and processes. Continuous improvement processes are very rare in American health care. That lack of process improvement is true primarily because the piecework payment model we use to buy care today generally prevents caregivers who improve care from realizing any benefit for their care site or their care business unit when care improvements are performed. The piecework payment model we use to buy care actually almost always penalizes caregivers for making care better or more efficient. That is a highly perverse impact. It needs to be understood. That real-world impact of that payment model seriously inhibits continuous improvement use in care delivery. Care sites do not do the work that is needed to eliminate duplicate tests for any given patient when each and every test generates a fee and when eliminating the test eliminates that fee -- with no reward of any kind for the care site that does the reengineering that eliminates the test. No business ever reengineers against its own self-interest. So the piecework payment approach inhibits care process improvement, and it also creates very rigid approaches to care.

Kaiser Permanente, by contrast, is not paid for care by the piece. Fees do not dictate care at Kaiser Permanente. The fact that the Kaiser Permanente care system is liberated from fees has been very useful in putting together the care delivery infrastructure and the entire array of care processes for patients that are much more patient focused instead of being fee-schedule focused.

The standard Medicare, Medicaid, and private insurance fee schedules that determine eligible care in other care settings do not define or limit care at Kaiser Permanente. That is a very different way of looking at care delivery design and opportunities. Those standard insurance fee schedules actually create rigid patterns of care for care sites in this country. Other care systems and care sites that are paid only by the piece usually only do the exact work that is listed on those insurer-approved fee schedules. Those schedules define a limited, rigid, and inflexible list of services.

Asthma patients, for example, can often benefit significantly when a nurse can call the patient to be sure the patient is refilling their prescriptions. The nurses can also coach each patient on effective early intervention approaches. That work by nurses can help reduce the number of asthma crises significantly. That fact has been proven repeatedly in several care settings. That proactive work is not done in most fee-based care settings, however, because having a nurse call a patient to coordinate needed care is not listed on the approved set of billable services for most payers. So instead of having children across the country who have fewer asthma crises, we have far too many children who end up in the emergency room actually going through the misery of a painful and terrifying asthma crisis that could have been prevented with proactive care approaches.

WE GET WHAT WE PAY FOR

The irony of that situation, of course, is that each and every one of those emergency care expenses that are needed for those asthma patients who are in a personal care crisis are all listed on the approved fee schedule. The caregivers are paid for that crisis care. Those very expensive sets of crisis response care services happen in great numbers across this country. They generate a lot of revenue. Nurse phone calls to patients to prevent asthma attacks are not on the approved fee schedule, however, so those nurse calls are rare.

The basic truth is pretty simple.

We get what we pay for. As noted earlier, in a well-structured, patient-centered medical home, the homes are paid a lump sum for multiple services. That lump sum cash flow per patient can liberate the care sites from that fee schedule for at least some services. Some level of lump sum payment per patient usually is used in those new team care settings -- and those lump sum payments can fund those kinds of nurse calls and proactive follow-up visits and contacts with the patients. Those lump sum payments can also fund e-visits between doctors and patients that are usually not reimbursed by the standard insurance fee schedule.

So medical homes and accountable care organizations that sell care as a package will be able to design their care and their information flow around the patient, and not just around the fee schedule. Those ACOs and medical homes can use nurses, electronic care connections, and much more flexible care approaches to meet patient needs.

Fourteen HIV Care Steps Not on a Medicare Fee Schedule

Multiple examples have shown that care can be a lot better when care processes are freed from fee-schedule rigidity.

At Kaiser Permanente, the care delivery strategy and approach that has reduced HIV deaths to less than half of the national average[146] has 14 steps in the most current care process that do not show up on a Medicare, Medicaid, or standard insurance company fee schedule.[147] Those 14 steps are patient-focused, nonbillable, nonfee-schedule activities that help create much better care outcomes for those HIV patients.

There is no "CPT" code for those services. If Kaiser Permanente only did the specific HIV treatment steps for those patients that are listed on the approved Medicare fee schedule -- and limited care to that fee schedule list of services -- the death rate for those patients could double. Twice as many people die today in the other care settings in America that are paid only by the piece for that care.

HIV isn't the only example of patient-focused care and better care that can result from the care team not being confined to a fee schedule. Kaiser Permanente has also reduced broken bones for seniors by over a third.[148] That is extremely important, life-saving work. A high percentage of older seniors who break bones die within a year. That work to prevent broken bones can be extremely important work for low income patients who don't have the resources to deal with the long term expenses for themselves and their families that can be created by a broken bone. Preventing those breaks is important work to do. Again -- six of the nine steps that are currently done to reduce the number of broken bones also do not show up on the Medicare or Medicaid fee schedule.[149] Those fee-schedule constraints dictate care in most care settings, and they are a reality we need to understand if we want to improve care.

Those defined fee-schedule approved service lists that are created and administered by Medicare, Medicaid, and by typical insurance companies generally restrict the delivery of care to a fairly rigid set of services. Those lists limit care, and they can badly cripple and even kill continuous improvement processes in American care sites.

REENGINEERING PROCESSES RARELY HAPPEN IN HEALTH CARE

Health care is almost alone in not using reengineering tools to improve processes and create efficiencies.

Reengineering processes have made huge improvements in both products and services in other multiple industries. Reengineering, by contrast, is a rare occurrence in health care. It is rare in health care because really well done reengineering processes often simplify whatever approach is being reengineered. As noted earlier, when you simplify anything in a piecework payment model, you run the risk of eliminating a billable piece for the caregiver from the overall care delivery process. Losing a billable piece from the process simply and purely reduces revenue. As noted earlier, no industry ever reengineers against its own self-interest. Health care follows that same path. Also, as noted earlier, even something as simple as eliminating duplicate tests between various care sites that are seeing the exact same patient is unlikely to happen in most care settings simply because each reduction of a duplicate service will reduce the revenue for that duplicating care site by the full payment amount they receive to do that particular service. When a scan can generate a 500- to 1,000-dollar invoice,[150] eliminating a scan to use the exact same test already done for that patient at another site simply reduces the revenue for that scan from the second site.

Again -- if the new ACOs are well-designed, and if they are set up to have a bundled payment of some kind for all needed care, and if the ACO business units are freed by their payers from the tyranny of a rigidly defined piecework cash flow -- then health care reengineering processes could flourish and thrive, and care improvement operational gains as basic as eliminating purely duplicate tests could be significantly encouraged.

LAB TEST RESULTS CAN GO DIRECTLY TO PATIENTS WITH NO REDUCTION IN CAREGIVER REVENUE

The number of unnecessary duplicate tests done at Kaiser Permanente today is tiny -- both because there is no additional revenue inside Kaiser Permanente for each test and because Kaiser Permanente has set up a computerized data flow support system that lets each test that is done for each patient be permanently stored in an electronic form and instantly available to every relevant caregiver who needs it in real time.

Likewise, a lab test result that is done at Kaiser Permanente goes directly from the laboratory to the medical record and also goes to the doctor who ordered the test. Processes for data flow relative to lab test results are much improved. It used to sometimes take days to get basic information from the lab to the caregivers and then to the patient. That work is now done in real time -- with the test results now ideally going to the caregiver instantly as each test is completed. For most basic outpatient tests at Kaiser Permanente, the lab results are usually also sent directly to the patient at the same time those lab results go to the physician. Kaiser Permanente patients received over 30 million lab results directly and on their personal computers and their smartphones last year.[151]

The payment model of being paid for an entire package of care made that whole, very convenient information flow to patients easy to do.

Why does being paid by the package instead of being paid by the piece make that type of direct information flow about lab tests more likely to happen?

Cash flow is the answer.

In standard fee-based care settings, the primary care doctors can usually bill for an additional office visit when the patients return to the doctor's office to get their lab tests. Those fees charged to the patients for those visits can run from 100 to 200 or more dollars per visit. When each of the patients who had the lab tests done comes back to the clinic and to the doctor's office to receive their lab results in person, that can generate a significant amount of cash for the care site.

At Kaiser Permanente, the lab results are still given to the patient in person by the doctor when there is a medical need for the visit with the doctor, but those visits with the doctor are not scheduled just to generate a bill for the care site. Most lab results go to the patient -- with a clear explanation of their significance -- and the patients do not need to return to the clinic to get the results in-person and onsite.

Being paid by the package and not by the piece clearly creates a whole range of care options and care delivery approaches that do not exist when insurance companies define each of the pieces of care that will generate a payment and keep those lists very rigid over time. Nearly a third of the care and care support resources that are used today inside Kaiser Permanente medical sites to support patient care are spent on services that would not trigger a Medicare, or Medicaid, or standard insurance company fee payment if Kaiser Permanente were to bill one of those payers for those services.

Kaiser Permanente has now invested billions of dollars in computerizing all aspects of the care data flow.[152] Kaiser Permanente did that work without worrying about whether or not any piece of care that would be supported by the new care systems would be billable. Everything relating to care data is now electronic. Imaging is done digitally. The entire medical record is electronic. Care reminders and care prompts are done electronically for both caregivers and patients.

One internal Kaiser Permanente care support system -- The Outpatient Safety Net -- is a highly complex computer program that scans the files looking for gaps in the fabric of needed care for Kaiser Permanente patients. That safety net data screening identifies specific care needs -- like needed but current follow-up visits for early-detection aneurysm patients. Or looking to see if patients who need some level of chronic care medication have, in fact, done their needed basic prescription refills.

Those care support systems have improved care.

The growing amount of number-one quality and number-one safety scores in the country on multiple care quality and care functionality issues that have been achieved by Kaiser Permanente caregivers isn't accidental or coincidental. It is entirely intentional. Computer support systems help both patients and care teams remember the right next steps for care, and then those systems help track whether or not those care steps were achieved. The extremely high level of blood pressure control that was mentioned in Chapter Two isn't accidental; nor is the high level of colon cancer detection. Overall, use of the new electronic care support tools is a learning process. Those systems are continuously improving. Flexible process design happens. Those care improvement steps are all being done without worrying about whether or not each and every piece of work will trigger a payment from an authorized fee schedule. There is no fee for tracking to see if newly diagnosed patients are filing their prescription, and there is no fee for running computer scans or to see if patients are doing follow-up care. There is no fee for coaching HIV patients on persistent medication compliance. But lives are saved -- and money is saved -- because those processes exist and do what they are intended to do.

SIX GUIDELINES THAT CAN HELP ANCHOR ACCOUNTABLE CARE

So Kaiser Permanente is already a model for accountable care. ACOs that are figuring out how to succeed in the new care delivery approach and cash flow model can and should look to Kaiser Permanente for some approaches that work well to meet those goals.

Those newly forming ACOs might find it useful to know that the basic accountable care process at Kaiser Permanente has made extensive use of six key guidelines. The six key guidelines should be extremely relevant and useful to anyone who is trying to improve overall care in an organizational setting. Those guidelines are of particular value to anyone who is trying to reduce the disparities in care that exist today between various ethnic and racial groups, because each of those guidelines tees up approaches and tools that can directly help reduce care disparities. The use of those guidelines has helped reduce care disparities at Kaiser Permanente.

The six key guidelines are:
1) All, All, All
2) Make the right thing easy to do
3) Continuously improve
4) Focus on the patient

5) Create available and transparent data

6) Be Us -- Eliminate Disparities

Many of the new care systems that are being established in other care settings could benefit significantly by using some or all of those same six guidelines for both planning and operations.

Those six guidelines are worth understanding because they did not happen in a vacuum. They did not come into being through theoretical, academic, externally created research. They are all working, functional guidelines that steer operational thinking and care improvement, and they all evolved through and with the care improvement agenda in place at Kaiser Permanente.

The first guideline is very basic. Guideline one is to have all of the information about each patient.

1) ALL/ALL/ALL

All, All, All is a very basic and foundational systems development guideline that all of America could and should follow as the new care systems are being created. All, All, All means all of the data about all of the patients all of the time. All of the key Kaiser Permanente systems, processes, and data flows have been built around that guideline, building on a patient-focused, patient-centered, and inclusive database for each patient -- with the functional and operational goal of all of those processes aimed at having each patient's data available in real time to the caregiver at the point of care.

If you understood care delivery, that guideline seems logical -- even simplistic. But the truth is that far too many other care settings today actually build their data infrastructure around their billing processes or around their actual physical care sites, rather than building their overall data planning and data flow around patients. Having site-specific data isn't entirely wrong. Having care-site relevant data can be a good thing -- but site-limited data is woefully and painfully inadequate as an overall data strategy. If caregivers only have patient data stored by site, then the data for each patient will be in splinters that are separated, segregated, and inadequate for care support. Data files that are defined and set up only by each of the patients' care sites is a really inadequate and dysfunctional way to design the data flows for care. The best way to design data storage and data linkages is to design the macro system to create electronic data about the care pieces for each patient so the computerized information from each element and site of care delivery constantly updates each patient's individual data file.

That all/all/all model works. That data organization creates a great tool. Care is better. The stroke death rate at Kaiser Permanente is down 40 percent in just a few years[153] because that full set of data exists for each patient and because the available care data is skillfully used by the care team and the caregivers.

This is a very good time for people in the care delivery world to think about that guideline.

Just about everyone in health care who isn't computerized now is planning to become computerized. Not everyone is planning to do their computerization in a way that creates a data focus that is built on each patient. Many sites who have already implemented electronic records only computerized their own site-specific data, and those care sites can't link their own data to other caregivers who are caring for the same patients. As noted earlier, that is a deeply inferior and badly flawed data model. That splintering isn't necessary, and it is highly dysfunctional.

So the advice point on that issue is this -- the rest of health care should not be setting up data projects or data use approaches that do not result in all/all/all data sharing for each patient. All/all/all works, and it should be the core of the system design and implementation efforts that are being done across all care sites -- particularly the ones who want to succeed as ACOs or function as medical homes. That work is very much needed if we want to reduce care delivery disparities and close care gaps in America.

2) MAKE THE RIGHT THING EASY TO DO

The second piece of advice is -- make the right thing easy to do.

Making the right thing easy to do is another very basic care mantra used at Kaiser Permanente that can and should be used by accountable care organizations and patient-centered medical homes across the country.

In the management of complex organizations, it can be very useful to have some basic underlying guidelines that function as the underpinnings of both strategic and operational thinking. "Make the Right Thing Easy to Do" is a basic guideline that serves that purpose for a wide range of issues at Kaiser Permanente. That guideline is used as a compass and a guidepost for figuring out how to deal with an entire array of functional situations -- including systems design, process development, and care infrastructure use.

The guideline has two key and highly important parts. The first part is to figure out the "right thing" to do for any given situation. The second part is to figure out how to make that "right thing" easy to do. When that two-part process is done well, it is immensely powerful and highly effective. Having all patient data available for caregivers is obviously a right thing to do, for example. The challenge for the systems people who follow that overall guidance is to figure out how to make access to that data easy to do. Likewise, having the best medical science available to caregivers is obviously a "right thing" to do. For most of the caregivers in the world, having consistent access to best medical science is not only not easy to do -- it is often impossible to do. Literally impossible. Medical science changes all the time. There are more than 80,000 medical journal articles published every year.[154] No individual doctor on the planet can read all of the relevant journals and still have time to see patients.

The Institute of Medicine (IOM) has recognized that for many care delivery situations, the current care practices and approaches of the caregivers are not based on the best available information.[155] The IOM now has a taskforce set up whose goal is to have 90 percent of the care delivered in this country based on best medical science by 2020.[156] The level of evidence-based care being done in this country is well below that 90-percent goal today.[157]

Kaiser Permanente recognized that the problem of making sure all caregivers have access to current and relevant medical information does exist. Kaiser Permanente believes that having access to that key information for every caregiver is very much "The Right Thing to Do."

So the challenge was -- how can that need to have access to medical science and to information about best care become easy to do for the caregivers of Kaiser Permanente?

How did Kaiser Permanente make scientific data access for caregivers easy to do?

The answer is elegant and simple.

Kaiser Permanente created an electronic medical library. The library is easily accessible. The library has in it all of the basic medical textbooks, hundreds of thousands of journal articles, and more than 2,500 best practice care protocols.[158] The care protocols are based on the best thinking of expert teams of caregivers who have looked systematically at the best medical science. The electronic medical library is available 24 hours a day, 7 days a week for all Kaiser Permanente caregivers. The library is even accessible by caregivers remotely using their smartphones or computers.

It is possible that no other major care team in the world has access to current medical science that is as complete, useful, and entirely functional as the data that is available today to the Kaiser Permanente care team. The electronic library has gone through several major enhancements that make it continuously easier to use. A standing committee of caregivers works on improving the system. An entire team of caregivers continuously refreshes the content and the science in the library. The research in the library is current because a dedicated, full-time team of medical experts reads through the research developed elsewhere in the world to find the nuggets and the key learnings that can be used to enhance the quality of care delivery at Kaiser Permanente.

Having access to the best medical science is the right thing to do. Embedding that science in an electronic library makes that right thing easy to do. The electronic library currently gets used roughly 1 million times every month by the care team.[159]

Other caregivers in this country need that same model. All of the organizations who are creating ACOs should be working on building or buying their own access to a functioning electronic medical library. Care consistency and best care are hard to do without electronic medical library tools of one kind or another.

MAJOR DIFFERENCES EXISTED IN THE DEATH RATE FOR STROKE PATIENTS

That entire "make the right thing easy to do" process also works well for stroke patient care. The stroke care improvement process was triggered in part by important research that was done on stroke deaths that happened inside Kaiser Permanente hospitals. Kaiser Permanente does a lot of research. Kaiser Permanente researchers currently publish over 1,200 articles each year in various medical journals.[160] One of the Kaiser Permanente research projects looked at the electronic medical record database for a couple million patients to study hospitalized stroke patients. The stroke study identified a very powerful link that existed between the use of the prescription drugs called statins and the death rate for hospitalized stroke patients. The researchers learned that there was a huge impact on the death rate for stroke patients -- depending on whether or not the stroke patients in the hospitals received statins. The death rate differences were significant.

The study learned that when hospitalized stroke patients were not given statins while they were hospitalized, the death rate for those patients was 11 percent. But when those same hospitalized stroke patients were given statins, the death rate dropped to 6 percent.[161]

So the researchers who were using the new electronic Kaiser Permanente database to look at stroke deaths identified from that vast array of data that the death rate for hospitalized stroke patients could be cut almost in half by giving the stroke patients statins while they were in the hospital. That was very important information. Cutting the death rate for stroke patients in half is obviously an important thing to do.

CHART – 4.1   **FOR ILLUSTRATIVE PURPOSES ONLY**

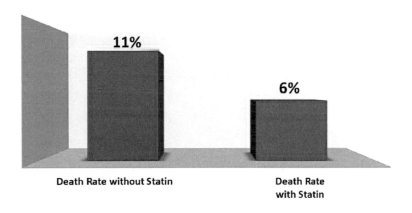

Overall Stroke Mortality Rate

11%

6%

Death Rate without Statin   Death Rate
with Statin

Source: Inpatient statin use predicts improved ischemic stroke discharge disposition. Kano O, Iwamoto K, Ikeda K, Iwasaki Y. Neurology. 2012 Dec 4; 79(23):2294.

The researchers also learned that for the stroke patients who survived, the percentage of patients who went home from the hospital either undamaged or lightly damaged was also significantly better for the patient group who received the statins.

That was an incredibly powerful learning. It was possible to do that learning only because Kaiser Permanente has put the electronic medical records in place for all patients that can be used to make that kind of research and learning "easy to do."

Under the rubric, "Make The Right Thing Easy To Do" -- medical research is obviously very much a right thing to do. Having a database that makes important medical research "easy to do" is even better.

That extremely important learning about cutting the death rate in half for those stroke patients would have been almost impossible to do in a research environment that had to use both pure paper medical records for all patients and small data pools.

Interestingly, cutting the stroke death rate by almost half for all stroke patients, on average, wasn't the most stunning learning that occurred as part of that particular research project. The most stunning data point resulted from the fact that the researchers also looked at the death rates in the hospital for the people who had strokes who had been taking statins before they were hospitalized for their strokes. That information about prior use of statins came from a different part of the electronic medical record. The researchers learned that for those stroke patients who had been taking statins before they were hospitalized and who then continued on with the use of statins while they were in the hospital, the death rate dropped to 5 percent.[162] Five percent is a very low number. Because Kaiser Permanente has the complete medical records for every patient electronically, the researchers could know which patients had been taking statins before being hospitalized.

In other research settings -- and particularly in any research settings where paper medical records are used as the database -- the analysts doing the research on those patients who died in the hospital typically would have no way of knowing any of that information about any prior use of statins by those patients.

That 5-percent number was the good news. There was also bad news. The bad news was that if the stroke patient had been taking statins before being hospitalized, and if the statins were then discontinued while the patient was hospitalized -- the death rate for those patients jumped to 23 percent.[163]

Twenty-three is a very big percentage. That is a high rate of death. That is incredibly important information. It is particularly important information for any patients who suffer strokes who have been currently taking statins. That number of stroke patients who take statins today is in the millions across the country. For those patients, the research shows that their chances of dying is roughly 1 in 20 if their statins are continued; and their chances of dying is roughly 1 in 4 if the statins are discontinued.[164]

CHART – 4.2   FOR ILLUSTRATIVE PURPOSES ONLY

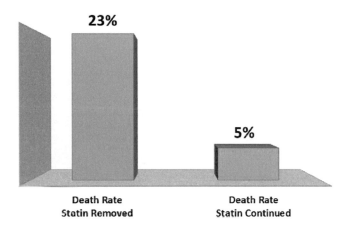

Stroke Mortality Rate -- Prior Statin Users

23%

5%

Death Rate
Statin Removed

Death Rate
Statin Continued

Source: Inpatient statin use predicts improved ischemic stroke discharge disposition. Kano O, Iwamoto K, Ikeda K, Iwasaki Y.
Neurology. 2012 Dec 4; 79(23):2294.

So what did Kaiser Permanente do with that extremely important stroke death rate information? How did Kaiser Permanente
make the right thing easy to do? The right thing to do for the stroke
patients was clearly identified.

As a first distribution point and an important communications approach, that piece of research was published in a highly
respected, fully refereed medical journal. The journal of Neurology
then shared that research finding with the world through their
normal distribution approaches. So Kaiser Permanente shared that
new piece of information with as many other caregivers as possible who might be treating stroke patients through publishing that
important piece of research in that highly respected and well read
medical journal.

That journal-publication approach is not, however, a perfect
information distribution system. Some other caregivers in multiple other care sites may have read that journal article, but very
many other caregivers who treat stroke patients every day do not
read that particular journal and did not read that particular article.

Nearly 80,000 other medical journal articles about various research topics were published that year. [165] Obviously, not every journal article gets read by every caregiver. For starters, it is clear that not all caregivers who treat stroke patients subscribe to that journal -- so if that was the only learning tool used to distribute that piece of information, it would not have helped all of the patients who would have benefited from that knowledge.

Inside Kaiser Permanente, both that journal article and the related research were added to the Kaiser Permanente electronic medical library. That was a first communications step inside Kaiser Permanente. In addition, a team of neurological experts analyzed the research, checked out the findings, and then developed a recommended Kaiser Permanente stroke treatment protocol that incorporated that information into the current guidelines.

So, to help make use of that important piece of research information about stroke patients easy to do, a medical best practices protocol including that science was developed, and the protocol was then distributed to Kaiser Permanente caregivers through the Kaiser Permanente electronic medical library.

As noted earlier, most other caregivers in the world do not have an electronic medical library -- so the truth is that relatively very few other caregivers outside of Kaiser Permanente actually received or learned about that piece of information about stroke patients.

That was not, however, the total use of that key piece of information about stroke care inside Kaiser Permanente. That library still needs to be accessed by a caregiver to have an impact on care. There is another level of care support tool inside Kaiser Permanente that can take the learning process one step further. As noted earlier, Kaiser Permanente owns and operates more than three dozen hospitals.[166] In the hospitals that are owned and operated by Kaiser Permanente, that extremely important piece of information about life-saving stroke treatment was also added to the recommended "order set" that is used in the hospitals by the caregivers at the point of care for each stroke patient. "Order sets" are a key functional and very useful care support tool. They help caregivers make right care easy to do. To make the right thing easy to do for this particular information, that highly important information about recommended "orders" for stroke patients appears on a screen in the hospital for the doctor to review exactly at the point in time when the Kaiser Permanente doctor is treating a stroke patient.

In other hospitals and other care settings, a stroke patient who had been taking statins before their stroke has to hope that their doctors might have seen that research article. The patients in other care sites also have to hope that their doctor might remember to make use of that information for them at that moment in time. Human memory -- simple mental recollection -- is the primary care quality support tool that is used for that kind of medical science reminder in the vast majority of all non-Kaiser Permanente care settings. Memory -- many studies have shown -- is an imperfect and often undependable quality safeguard, and sheer and pure memory obviously isn't functionally optimal as an anchor of any care or safety process.

By contrast -- at Kaiser Permanente -- the basic research about stroke deaths was read, understood, incorporated into care guidelines, and then that valuable information was also built systematically into the computerized care "prompts" that are used at the point and the site of care to remind the caregivers of that information at the exact time when making that "right thing" easy to do was most important to the patient. Making the right thing easy to do clearly increases the likelihood that the right thing will be done.

Each of those pieces -- computerized care protocols and computerized recommended order sets should be considered by the people who are putting ACOs in place in various care settings. That could be a good time to at least begin that work.

Making the right thing easy to do is also why Kaiser Permanente has developed an extensive, award-winning, mail-based prescription refill program. The new tool kit allows for prescription refills to be either triggered or ordered on the patient's computer or smartphone.

Why does that fit the category of making the right thing easy to do?

If you want to help prevent heart attacks, asthma attacks, CHF attacks, and strokes, the right thing to do is to get the patients who are individually at the most risk for those conditions to take their medications. In that context, making the right thing very easy to do for the patient who is refilling their prescriptions is a very good care support strategy.

That approach works. Kaiser Permanente has some of the highest prescription refill rates in the nation[167] -- and Kaiser Permanente is seeing reduced numbers of both strokes and heart attacks.

It is much more convenient -- significantly easier for most patients to do -- for the patient to get their prescriptions by mail rather than driving to a pharmacy to get a refill. Last year, Kaiser Permanente filled more than 30 million prescriptions by mail.[168] The actual, pure energy savings that resulted from those patients not having to drive to a pharmacy to get their drugs actually has its own environmental protection value.

Likewise -- to make the right thing easy to do -- Kaiser Permanente has set up approaches that allow patients to have e-visits with their caregivers. ACOs and medical homes can also both learn from that model. It works well. Patients like the model, and caregivers find it extremely useful. With secure messaging, email visits between patients and physicians can both supplement and replace face-to-face visits for many care situations. Kaiser Permanent had roughly 12 million of those e-visit connections with patients and physicians last year.[169] That information sharing and that direct-patient dialogue with the physician would have required a face-to-face visit in almost all of those piecework-reimbursed care settings. The patient would need a face-to-face meeting with a caregiver in a medical office site to get that e-visit information flow and that physician dialogue in almost all other care settings. Each of those face-to-face visits in the fee-based care settings would also have triggered an office visit fee -- ranging from a hundred dollars to a couple hundred dollars.[170] Because Kaiser Permanente doesn't bill for care by the piece, there was no revenue loss to Kaiser Permanente for creating those highly convenient, patient/physician electronic interactions. E-visits clearly make the right thing easy to do for patients.

Again -- looking at the rest of the world -- when millions of additional low income and minority people will get insurance of one kind or another for the first time at the beginning of next year, having care sites available to those patients that can offer e-connections for patients instead of just face-to-face visits, would clearly be a very good thing for many newly insured patients. The logistical conveniences of those visits could be particularly useful for low income patients. Low income people often face transportation difficulties. Those difficulties can be mitigated for many people by having some care contacts with their care teams be done electronically rather than just having all care contacts happening as face-to-face visits in the physician's physical care sites. That would make the right thing easy to do for those patients -- and making the right thing easy to do is a highly useful guideline for the new ACOs and medical homes to follow.

3) CONTINUOUSLY IMPROVE

Continuous improvement is another key guideline at Kaiser Permanente. The third Kaiser Permanente guideline that should be relevant and useful to ACOs and medical homes as this country begins to reorganize the way we both deliver and buy care in this country is to "continuously improve." Continuous improvement is an approach to care that has huge value. Dealing with the issues of care differences and care disparities is much more likely to be successful in the context of continuous improvement for care delivery.

Continuous improvement is now a core philosophy for Kaiser Permanente planning functionality and operations. Most of health care in this country is delivered today in care sites that are heavily focused on maintaining, protecting, and preserving their status quo. Process change is rare. Very few care sites in America have set up formal processes and built the skill sets that are needed to achieve continuous improvement. Continuous improvement, done well, involves gathering data, measuring results, and taking appropriate steps in a formal, systematic way to improve the results of any process.

Continuous improvement -- done really well -- reaches beyond simply improving current processes and extends to inventing new approaches and new processes where a significant level of change is needed to continuously improve care delivery.

For hospital-acquired pressure ulcers, for example, the continuous improvement process started with measuring the number of ulcers that were happening. Once the initial measures were identified, teams of caregivers began figuring out ways of reducing the number of those ulcers. Standard care approaches -- like continuous inspection by caring nurses of the skin health of each and every high-risk patient -- were developed, applied, implemented, tested for effectiveness, and then continuously improved. Best practices were developed and shared. As noted earlier in this book, the percentage of patients in Kaiser Permanente hospitals with those ulcers dropped over time from nearly 4 percent of the patients to less than 1 percent.[171] Improvements in treatments, skin care medications and even buildings and equipment were all added to that approach over time in a process of functional continuous improvement.

Continuous improvement is more than goal-setting.

The functional continuous improvement approach that is used by Kaiser Permanente for care improvement is not just to set a goal for some area of performance, achieve the goal, and then declare victory. The approach used at Kaiser Permanente in most settings is to set a direction for improvement and then continuously improve. Pressure ulcers are a good example. Continuous improvement for that particular category of care has worked to the point where several Kaiser Permanente hospitals have not had one single stage 2 pressure ulcer in over a year.[172]

Again, the fact that Kaiser Permanente sells care by the package -- very much like the new ACOs hope to do -- instead of just selling care by the piece, creates a very different business model. In those piecework payment settings, where care is sold by the piece and not by the package, reducing the number of pressure ulcers to zero could actually result in a significant reduction in hospital revenue.

However -- and this is the important point to recognize -- if those hospitals were paid a flat ACO payment that was level and fixed per patient, that lump sum payment approach does not create any new revenue for a hospital when patients get those ulcers. Continuous improvement processes could become a functional reality in those ACO settings -- and the number of additional hospitals in other care settings who would also be able to achieve zero ulcers for their patients would probably increase significantly. Continuous improvement clearly works best when that care is sold by the package and not by the piece.

Continuous-improvement thinking and approaches can be seen in all of the overall continuously improving results that were shown on all of the performance charts in Chapter Two of this book. Care obviously got better for each condition, each year. The performance levels did not get to a point where the fact that Kaiser Permanente had the best levels in the country in some areas was good enough. "Best" is not the goal of continuous improvement. The goal of continuous improvement is to do better than best. Getting better is the key and ongoing goal. A widely stated adage inside Kaiser Permanente that functions as a subset and a corollary to the overall continuous improvement agenda is for Kaiser Permanente to be, "The Best at Getting Better."

Being "The Best at Getting Better," is also a very self-reinforcing goal. That is another important learning for the new ACOs and medical homes. When people believe that being the best at getting better is their operational goal, that goal liberates people to first figure out new ways of doing things and then to figure out even better ways of doing things. Again, the fact that Kaiser Permanente is not confined to only delivering the care that is defined by the pieces of care that are listed on a standard Medicare fee schedule helps immensely with flexibility and creativity relative to continuous improvement.

The current fee schedule for most payers deals with various aspects of care process flexibility in some obviously perverse ways. Cutting pressure ulcers to less than 1 percent of patients does not have one single fee-schedule trigger for a typical, standard, insurance-company-approved payment procedure scale. Having the nurses in each hospital carefully checking the skin of every patient repeatedly is a wonderful and highly effective thing to do -- but that work by those nurses does not generate a fee for any of the piecework-based care sites when the nurses do that work. Pressure ulcers can obviously create revenue from private insurers in a piecework setting. The work done to prevent pressure ulcers does not create revenue from those private insurers in those same settings. That is a bad way to buy care. The inherent perversity of that payment model is fairly obvious to anyone who looks closely at how we usually buy care in this country today.

There are 1.7 million Americans who get infections in hospitals every year that they did not have on the day they were admitted to the hospital. [173] Those infections can each trigger a lot of money for the hospitals where the patients were infected. Hospitals are all very ethical. Hospital leaders are all good people. Hospital medical directors are all good people. No hospital in this country would ever give any patient an infection deliberately. Never. None. That does not happen. That will not happen. But when no one pays for all of the work that is needed to effectively prevent those infections, it is also true that the work needed to prevent those infections tends not to get done in too many places -- unless you happen to be in a care setting like Kaiser Permanente where the care is sold as a package and not by the piece.

As noted earlier, the good news is that the new ACOs are likely to put continuous improvement processes in place, and care safety programs in operation that will trigger both prevention and rapid and effective response work if the payment model is set up appropriately to reward the consequences of better care. That level of successful prevention work is entirely possible to do. As a proto-type ACO, Kaiser Permanente is proving today that it can be done.

The functional and operational approach that guides the care delivery infrastructure of this country needs to be continuous improvement -- not maximizing revenue streams and optimizing billing units.

4) Focus on the Patient

Focusing on the patient is the fourth guideline.

A major Kaiser Permanente guideline for planning, opera-tions, and systems design that also deserves to be understood and replicated in various settings is focusing on the patient. That guideline also ought to be incorporated into the founda-tional structure of the new ACOs and medical homes. Patient focus is a key planning guideline and a major objective of the care system at Kaiser Permanente. Patient focus also seems like an obvious goal to many people, but it is not how most health care systems and most care infrastructure pieces in this country are designed today. For many areas of functionality, most care settings are designed almost entirely around the business needs of the caregivers. Systems that exist are set up primarily to gen-erate bills, and those billing-based systems only keep track of the data about the actual pieces of care that were delivered to a given patient at that specific care site. Very few systems are set up to link with one another in any way when a given patient has multiple caregivers. Very few systems or processes are set up by care sites to provide any data other than the information that is needed at that specific care site to deliver the site-specific pieces of care and to generate and process an insurance claim. The data that does exist in those care sites is almost entirely focused on each piece of care that was delivered -- not on the actual patient.

At Kaiser Permanente, by contrast, because the overall Kaiser Permanente care system is responsible for the total care needs of a full population of patients, the database and data flow are both set up with the patient at the core. That is actually a very useful and functional way to organize care data.

As noted earlier, the foundation and the anchor for all care data at Kaiser Permanente is the patient. The medical records for each patient are computerized, and all data from all systems about the care for each patient flows to that medical record. The lab systems run their tests, generate their reports, and that report data then goes from the lab system to the doctor and also flows electronically into each patient's activated medical record. Diagnostic and treatment information are not kept in separate files at Kaiser Permanente that are splintered and segregated by medical specialty or by care site. All of that information from all of the tests, the labs, and the care sites is kept as a total, patient-focused package in each patient's medical record.

That is a very practical way to use and file data.

That patient focus means that all of the data needed by the care-giver is available when it is needed at the point of care. That data collection approach also means that the computer can screen each patient's data files to see if all needed tests were done -- or if the patient is current on their prevention and on their personal, early detection and early intervention agendas.

The computer can even do very sophisticated screenings to look for unmet care needs. That can be particularly useful when the goal is to close care gaps and end disparities in care. There is no possible way to do that kind of systematic care process improvement work without an electric medical record and without a data system that focuses on patient-specific data to identify care needs in a systematic way.

Some care systems and care sites who do implement electronic medical records for their own care business units put electronic records in place that are segregated by care site or by medical specialty. Both of those approaches are clearly inferior to an approach where the care delivery and the care data are focused on the patients and all patient data is accessible through a single tool for each patient.

5) DATA AVAILABILITY – DATA TRANSPARENCY

Data needs to be both transparent and available.

The fifth Kaiser Permanente guideline and systems design goal that should be understood and probably followed by other care sites that are trying to improve care is to create both data availability and data transparency inside the organization or care team. Data about care is a wonderful thing to have. As noted earlier, health care in this country tends to be almost data free. There actually are huge deficits relative to both data gathering and data sharing in American health care delivery. Most patient data tends to be both splintered and inaccessible. Comparisons of all kinds are functionally impossible. Most care sites do not even know their own success levels and their own mortality rates for multiple health conditions -- much less knowing how their own performance compares with other caregivers who are treating people with the same health conditions.

That data void is a problem because there are significant variations in care performance levels.

The truth is that your personal chances of dying from cancer can double or triple, based on the care site you use. When you look at the five-year survival rates for breast cancer, the very best care sites have about a 5 percent mortality rate, and the very worst care sites have more than a 15 percent average mortality rate.[174] The bar chart below shows four numbers. One bar is the most recent breast cancer mortality rate in rural Georgia. The second bar shows the breast cancer mortality rate for cancer patients in Atlanta, Georgia. The third bar shows the breast cancer survival rates -- on average -- in the various cancer sites that participate in the SEER national cancer reporting database that was mentioned earlier in this book.

The fourth bar on the chart shows the average five-year survival rate for breast cancer cases at Kaiser Permanente.

CHART – 4.3

FOR ILLUSTRATIVE PURPOSES ONLY

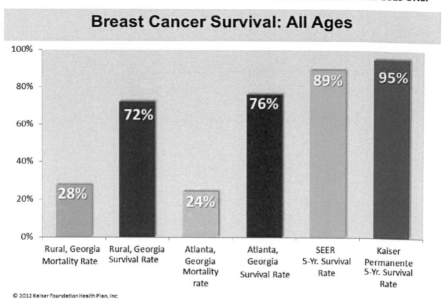

Breast Cancer Survival: All Ages

© 2012 Kaiser Foundation Health Plan, Inc.

There are some clear care disparities on this chart. Care is not the same everywhere. Care outcomes vary significantly. Too many caregivers do not even know how their outcomes for their own patients compare with the outcomes for patients at other care sites. It is hard for those sites to improve their care -- because they don't know how much improvement is possible. Patients should know what the potential survival rate differences are for key areas of care. In this particular case -- for cancer of the breast -- some of the major disparities for cancer survival rates are by geography and care site. Patients -- and particularly breast cancer patients -- need to know that these kinds of outcome differences exist.

Cancer isn't alone in having variable success levels for different care teams. The death rate varies by more than 60 percent for heart attacks between various hospitals.[175] For heart bypass surgery, the worst care sites have a death rate that is more than eight times higher than the death rate at the best care sites.[176]

GOOD INTENTIONS ARE NOT AS GOOD AS GOOD DATA

What is really unfortunate is that many of the low performing care sites have no clue about how badly they are doing. They have no clue because they do not have data. If those care sites sometimes do have some data, they often have only a snapshot piece of data. Single and isolated data points are not very valuable as the basis for any kind of continuous improvement activities for any care sites. Care can get a lot better when comparative data exists. Remember the sepsis care experience described earlier. The dozen hospitals that were listed on the sepsis mortality chart shown earlier, and shown again here, had no clue how well or badly they were each doing before the data was recorded.

CHART – 4.4

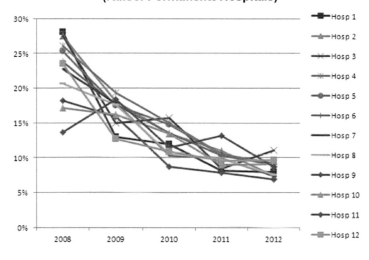

Basic Inpatient Mortality Among Patients with Sepsis
(Kaiser Permanente Hospitals)

© 2012 Kaiser Foundation Health Plan, Inc.

Before this data was gathered, all hospitals believed they were delivering great sepsis care.

The worst hospitals on this chart believed very sincerely, when this data was first gathered, that they were doing really good work with sepsis patients. The hospital teams were all very good people. They all knew very good approaches to sepsis care. They all knew the basic science of sepsis care. They were -- as a group -- extremely well-intentioned. It's hard to be better intentioned. But good intentions are not as good as good data when it comes to functionally saving lives.

The process of care improvement for sepsis deaths in those hospitals took more than data. It required transparency. To use that data really well, the hospitals first needed to share it with one another. If Hospital A only has the current data for Hospital A, there is no way of Hospital A knowing whether their performance is good or not good. Multiple data sources are needed to gain that insight. Comparisons are golden.

Sharing is also golden at multiple levels. The hospitals who had the lowest death rates for sepsis shared their best practices with the hospitals with lower success levels. That sharing process not only helped the poor performers -- it helped the good performers get better because they all learned from each other. Hiding data and not sharing data is not a good thing to do. A lot of people would literally be dead today if the 12 hospitals on this chart had hidden their data and not shared it with one another.

Sepsis is the number one cause of death in hospitals.[177] Cutting the death rate by two-thirds or more could have a large impact on overall hospital mortality rates in this country. We need all hospitals sharing their data about a wide range of mortality issues -- and care will get better when that happens.

In some ways, as noted earlier in this book, the most important success that results from the sepsis care improvement is that the patients who do survive in the best hospitals tend to be much less damaged than the patients who survive less effective sepsis care in the worst hospitals. Patients in the worst hospitals are much more likely to be damaged for life by their sepsis. That is another area of commonplace that can trigger life-long disparities by race and ethnicity that damage patients. That long term sepsis damage can be particularly debilitating for low income patients who have no financial resources to use to give themselves needed extra levels of support when they return badly damaged to their homes. There are significant subsequent disparities that happen at very basic economic levels when patients go home damaged by slow and inadequate sepsis care or by inferior and inadequate stroke care or pressure ulcer care.

We Need Data to Address Disparities

We will not be able to reduce disparities in this country if we don't have good data to let us know when disparities exist.

The key point of this section of the book is that we really do need good, solid, accurate, timely and actionable data about care performance -- and we need that data to be transparent between caregivers so we can make the kinds of informed decisions we need to make about continuously improving care across all populations. We very much need that data so we can reduce the disparities in care delivery that exist today. We need to define those disparities, understand them, identify where they happen, and take steps to mitigate and prevent them.

A major, recent study was released as -- "Predominately Black Hospitals Provide Poor Trauma Care."[178] The study showed that victims of trauma care were at much higher risk of dying if they were treated in hospitals that had a high number of Black patients. That level of performance needs to be corrected. Care in those hospitals will only improve when the care performance levels are visible to the caregivers and when the care processes in those care sites are systematically improved.

Kaiser Permanente has put together a database about care delivery that gathers that kind of data and uses it for those specific purposes. That approach can succeed. Care clearly gets better when that data use happens. The experiment that will determine whether or not data supported care improvement is good to do has been done. That approach is a good one, and it is obviously the right thing to do. The experiment of whether that entire database and systematic care improvement work can be used to prevent, alleviate, mitigate, and overcome the disparities that continue to exist in care delivery is a work in progress. It appears that progress is possible -- and we really need to learn from both our failures and our successes on those agendas.

6) Be Us -- Eliminate Disparities

The final Kaiser Permanente guideline that can be used to help American health care organizations and health plans address the issues of care disparities and care differences is to create an explicit and collective commitment for the care team to deliver the right care for all members of the patient population -- regardless of race, ethnicity, age, sexual alignment, or gender.

As you can see from the data that was shown earlier in this book -- with particular reinforcement from the care results that relate to HIV/AIDS patients and best care delivery -- it is important to make both care equity and care quality a key and explicit agenda of the care teams. It is important for care teams to think of all patients as being a collective part of who each care team is -- not seeing patients as separate sets of people who are defined by their race and ethnicity. It is a good thing to be inclusive in our thinking and to deal with all patients as being part of us -- included in our broad definition of who we are as caregivers and people.

That work of being inclusive is so important. That particular guidance is a separate chapter of this book. It is the next and final chapter.

Read on.

CHAPTER FIVE

WE NEED THE RIGHT VALUES AND THE RIGHT TOOLS TO CREATE THE RIGHT CARE

The achievements at Kaiser Permanente in reducing care gaps over the past couple of years for all groups of Kaiser Permanente patients that are described in this book are not accidental, and they are not insignificant. That work is far from perfect, but the truth is that those real-world, gap-reduction successes have been accomplished in the context of a large, integrated care system that is actually functionally accountable for the real-world health care needs of a very large and very diverse population of people.

As noted earlier, Kaiser Permanente is not doing its gap-reduction work in a small, isolated setting.

Kaiser Permanente serves 9 million patients.[179] Kaiser Permanente serves more patients than 40 states and 146 countries.[180] Kaiser Permanente has a patient population that is significantly more diverse than the country at large.[181] The Kaiser Permanente patient base is actually now more than half minority.[182] As the earlier chapters of this book demonstrated, Kaiser Permanente has been working hard to very explicitly identify areas where internal care differences and care disparities exist -- with the goal of eliminating any care gaps that exist inside Kaiser Permanente over a relatively short time frame.

That effort has had challenges and setbacks -- but it has over-whelmingly been successful -- and the continuous improvement commitment that was described in the last chapter is highly likely to be a factor in making those successes even better in the future.

The rest of the country can now look at the systems and the tools that have been built at Kaiser Permanente to do this work and can know that those systems make great logical sense and that the care improvement agenda and the gap-closing strategies actually work when those tools are in place and are used.

As noted earlier, those achievements have all been achieved by a staff that is one of the most diverse staffs in health care. The Kaiser Permanente staff is currently 58 percent minority.[183] The leadership and the Board of Kaiser Permanente are also both highly diverse.[184] Kaiser Permanente has managed to turn that staff-level diversity into functional synergy and into high levels of performance in multiple ways.

One of the more useful tools for accomplishing many of these goals has been an annual Diversity Conference that has been held at Kaiser Permanente for several decades. The Kaiser Permanente Diversity Conference brings together people to look at ways of pro-viding best care to a very diverse set of patients. For the last decade, one of the key topics every year at that conference has been a dis-cussion of the advantages that are created by having an organiza-tional sense of "Us."

In fact, one of the basic reasons for all of that operational and care improvement success has been a healthy sense of "Us" at Kaiser Permanente. It's actually important for almost any complex organization to have a clear internal sense of Us in order to increase the likelihood of organizational success. It's good to be Us.

Humans tend to divide the world into us and them and to treat people very differently based on whether someone is perceived to be an "Us" or perceived to be a "Them." The behavior differences can be significant.

We tend to be protective, supportive, nurturing, kind, and forgiving when we perceive someone else to be an Us. We tend to take care of people who are our an Us, and we are angry and protective when anyone else does damage to someone we perceive to be an Us.

By contrast, if someone is perceived to be a "Them," we are suspicious, antagonistic, distrustful, territorial, and even paranoid about the behavior of a Them. We discriminate against Them. We tend to stereotype and dehumanize Them. We too often feel no guilt or ethical discomfort when we do bad things to a "them."

Those are ugly and sad words, but those statements are far too often accurate and true.

The patterns of us/them behaviors that exist in many settings can be disruptive and divisive. Those unfortunate patterns have been seen repeatedly in many settings throughout human history. Look at the historical record. It is easy to see how us/them behaviors have caused people to behave in unfortunate ways in far too many instances.

"We" can do very bad things to "Them."

We enslave Them. We ethnically cleanse Them. We displace Them. And we far too often discriminate both legally and functionally against Them. In many traditional settings, we don't allow Them to marry our sons or daughters, and we often don't want Them in our community or in our neighborhood. People who have those destructive us/them values activated tend to resist the inclusion of whoever is perceived to be a Them in the workforce.

In too many instances, the care given to people perceived to be a Them can be truly horrible care. The German treatment of the Jews in the concentration camps by even the medical staff was a horrible us/them, guilt-free set of behaviors.

The medical world is obviously not immune to us/them behaviors.

The horrible Tuskegee experiment[185] of the last century where African Americans with syphilis were allowed to let the disease consume their bodies and kill the patients with no care delivery to save them was a horrible us/them guilt-free set of behaviors. Not giving painkillers to minority patients who are having heart attacks isn't as bad as denying all care to syphilis patients, but that behavior can spring from some of the same sorts of prejudicial beliefs.

We see those behaviors in many settings. Sometimes the group definition that activates the Us instincts is racial. Sometimes the group definition is tribal. Sometimes the us/them distinctions are either ethnic or cultural.

Family and clan identities can activate those instincts. Tribal identities create a sense of Us for some people and national identities can create a sense of Us for other people.

A shared set of values and a clear, collective identity in an organization setting can also activate a sense of Us.

Unfortunately, we humans can too easily fall prey to the negative side of those us/them beliefs and behaviors. The very good news is that we all have the ability to be an Us. The good news is that when we perceive people to be an Us, that perception of being an Us can activate the noble, caring, sharing aspects of our personalities and our behaviors.

As noted above, those sets of issues have been discussed at every Kaiser Permanente National Diversity Conference for over a decade. Creating a sense of us is a very useful and powerful thing for a care system to do, and it is very good to understand the impact of those instinctive emotions in health care settings and behaviors. It is very clear that there is great value in focusing on the behaviors and the processes that create a sense of collective and inclusive us.

That doesn't always happen in care settings in this country or anywhere else in the world.

Some of the disparities that exist today in care delivery are clearly caused by us/them-linked discriminatory behavior. Bias happens. Sometimes the bias is conscious and sometimes it is completely unconscious. When caregivers perceive their patients to be a Them, instead of Us, then the care given to those patients can too easily be discriminatory treatment approaches. As noted earlier, not giving painkillers to Black patients who are having heart attacks is a behavior where the caregivers are making discriminatory care choices that are based on a patient's race rather than making those care decisions based on each patient's actual care needs.

When children with autism who are Black or brown are more than 60 percent less likely to get referrals to specialty care even when those children are being seen in the same care system by the same primary care doctors[186] -- that is a form of us/them-centered biased behavior.

On the other hand, when a care team recognizes the universality of Us -- a human Us instead of a racial or ethnic Us -- then the care that is delivered by that care team can be done in ways that can reduce and eliminate disparities and create great care.

It is true that there are some times when some differences in care approaches are medically correct. The incredible work that has been done at Kaiser Permanente to end the differences in care results by race for I IIV patients was only possible because the caregivers and the care teams involved in that care clearly perceived all of the patients to be an Us and respected the racial and ethnic diversity of the patients at the same time.

Kaiser Permanente very deliberately works consistently to both create a sense of Us and to meet the needs of each patient as an individual human being -- not as a stereotype or a group representative, but as a person whose human needs are individually defined. That approach of recognizing differences and including everyone as a human Us results in better care for everyone.

As noted earlier, Kaiser Permanente holds an annual diversity conference. This conference is not a new thing. That conference has been happening for over 40 years. At that conference, hundreds of caregivers gather every year to learn the best ways of dealing with the issues that result from the various populations of patients. The caregivers share an overall commitment collectively to all of the patients. You can see from the session topics at that conference that the focus of that work is on both medical competence and cultural competence -- with sometimes controversial and challenging issues like unconscious bias clearly generically discussed and openly addressed.

The list of agenda items at last year's conference speaks for itself.

The first session was titled, "Diversity is One of Our Major Assets and Strengths."

The second talk was titled, "Is Excellent Good Enough?"

The third topic was, "A Road Map to Reducing Racial and Ethnic Health Disparities -- Evidence-Based, Game-Changing Strategies."

The fourth topic was, "From Theory to Practice -- Solutions at Kaiser Permanente."

Other topics that followed for the two-day conference included, "A World without Disparities -- Healing Healthcare Through Diversity and Inclusion."

Another agenda topic identified, "Community HIV/AIDS Game Changers."

Another topic was, "Leveraging Diversity."

There were sessions on education, community health, healthy behaviors, unconscious bias, and recognizing top performers for disparity reductions.

One topic was, "Advancing Diversity through the Discipline of Business Performance Management."

Another topic was, "Become a Weight of the Nation Activist in Your Community."

A session that was very powerful and effective was, "My Stories, My Expertise, My Voice -- Transgender Individuals and the Health Care System."

One side room at the conference was called an "Imaginarium." That room featured state-of-the-art technology tools that would be used to deliver care more effectively to diverse populations. One of the Imaginarium tools was a walking robot that could extend multicultural medical specialty expertise to actual hospital rounds remotely with a mobile medical robot.

The agenda for the next diversity conference will include topics intended to "Accelerate the Spread of Culturally Sensitive and Linguistically Effective Practices."

Another portion of the training will be focused on, "Creating High Workforce Engagement through Diverse, Inclusive Environments to Achieve High Productivity and Innovation."

It is clear from those agenda items that the high quality of care that exists across the entire multiracial patient population at Kaiser Permanente isn't accidental. That success in care delivery is the deliberate result of quality agendas that are focused on a wide range of issues that are relevant to a diverse patient base, and it is the result of a clear collaboration and collective alignment inside Kaiser Permanente of the value that can result for an organization from diversity.

Kaiser Permanente looks at the entire patient-base as Us -- a human Us -- and that diverse patient base is celebrated, appreciated, honored, respected, and well-served by caregivers who are also a "Human Us."

Kaiser Permanente also has one of the more successful labor management partnerships in the country -- and that partnership is anchored by a "Value Compass" that is centered on the patients that are served by the entire Kaiser Permanente care team.

The ongoing achievements of successful diversity practices inside Kaiser Permanente have been recognized by several external organizations. Kaiser Permanente has won the National DiversityInc. ranking as one of the best places to work for minority workers in the country.[187] Diversity MBA Magazine rated Kaiser Permanente as the best place to work for minority MBA holders.[188] Computerworld Magazine rated Kaiser Permanente one of the top two places to work in health care for minority IT employees.[189] The National Hispanic Chamber of Commerce recently added Kaiser Permanente to its diversity champion hall of fame.[190] Those distinctions and recognitions reflect the sense that Kaiser Permanente celebrates its diversity and embraces inclusion of all people from all groups as a way of life. The overall diversity agenda at Kaiser Permanente is far from perfect, and it is still in a state of learning -- but it is clearly moving in the right direction.

DEATH RATES ARE HIGHER AT BLACK HOSPITALS

As noted earlier, a recent study was covered in a major newspaper which said, "Death Rates Higher at Black Hospitals."[191]

The articles under those headlines had data showing significantly higher death rates at hospitals in this country that served primarily Black patients. There are a number of reasons why those negative outcomes exist. There is, however, no excuse for having lower standards of care for those hospitals. Care improvement is needed in each of those settings. That headline should never happen in this country.

Inside Kaiser Permanente, the death rates are obviously not higher at the hospitals that serve more Black patients. As you can see from the performance gap charts included earlier in this book, however, there are still differences in outcomes and care processes by race and ethnicity for a number of care areas inside the Kaiser Permanente care system. Those gaps are known. They are being addressed -- and they are closing. Recently, some Kaiser Permanente care sites have very successfully completely closed the gap among groups mentioned in Chapter Two of this book for hypertension. All of the other care sites at Kaiser Permanente are committed to bringing the full set of other gaps to closure over the next couple of years.

DISPARITY REDUCTION TAKES DATA, COMMITMENT, AND FULL EQUITY

For the rest of America to move in that same direction, we need the rest of health care to build the kinds of databased care support tools that exist today at Kaiser Permanente. There is no good reason for those tools not to be built and used in other care settings now that they have been invented and now that their value has been proven.

That disparities-reduction work in those other settings will depend on a care infrastructure and a care culture that is databased, transparent, directly committed to both continuous improvement and patient equity, and that is very directly patient-focused.

That progress is most likely to succeed in the context of a care team who sees itself as an inclusive Us and who knows and believes that the patients who are served by the care team are also an inclusive Us.

We Need Those Kinds of Successes to Happen Everywhere

For the rest of the country, we need to set up a situation where the kinds of care improvement wins that have been created at Kaiser Permanente across all racial and ethnic groups are possible everywhere -- regardless of the site of care. Tools are needed. Data is needed. We need to set up medical homes and ACOs that have clear data files for each patient and provide well-coordinated team care. New ACOs and medical homes are being created every day. We need all of those new ACO and medical home care settings to commit to continuous improvement approaches for care delivery for all of their patients.

To the extent that Medicaid becomes a program where the states decide to hire health plans or hire care systems to be their functioning Medicaid care infrastructure, it also would be the right thing to do to build the right purchasing specifications for those programs. The states should require the vendors they hire to deliver care under their Medicaid agenda to create the right levels of data transparency, team care, and continuously improving care as part of the purchasing criteria. That database for the Medicaid patients should be capable of detecting care disparities when they exist, and it should support the work needed to make the disparities disappear in a systematic way

We need to put in place a business model for care that allows the care delivery infrastructure to do intelligent and effective care process reengineering without going bankrupt and to reduce care disparities with the full support of the tools needed to do that work.

INTELLIGENT CHANGE IS THE RIGHT AGENDA

Change is needed. Change is inevitable. Intelligent change is the right agenda for the new array of opportunities we have right in front of us.

We clearly do need to reduce health care disparities in this country. We should not have a death rate for patients that increases by 50 percent or more for a given condition, based on the race and ethnicity of the patient. We need to keep track of the care delivered to each set of patients to achieve that disparity reduction agenda -- and we need to set a target for ourselves as a nation set on ending the more than four, full-year life expectancy gap[192] that exists today between Americans and African Americans. We need to shrink that gap by improving the life expectancy for African Americans.

It is time to do the work needed to make that happen. This book points out what several major elements of that work should be.

None of that will happen if our primary strategy for ending disparities is wishful thinking and goodwill. We will not close those care gaps with good intentions. Gaps can be closed, but we will need to work hard with real tools to make that happen.

We need to use all of our resources and all of the new tools well to achieve the goal that is clearly described in the title of this book. It's time for us to "End Racial, Ethnic, and Cultural Disparities in American Health Care."

We spend more money on health care than anyone in the world by a huge percentage. We very much deserve best care for all of us, for all of those dollars that we are spending.

The time to do that work is now.

Be well.

Kaiser Permanente Awards and Recognitions for Quality, Service, Creativity and Functionality

2013

❖ "Foundation of the Year" Award. Gov. Edmund G. Brown Jr.'s 2013 Volunteer Service Awards. June 2013.

❖ Twenty-nine Environmental Excellence Awards. Practice Greenhealth. May 31, 2013.

❖ Platinum Award for Best Employer for Healthy Lifestyles. National Business Group on Health. May 22, 2013.

❖ Leapfrog Award for Kaiser Permanente Hospitals Rated Among Safest in the Nation. The Leapfrog Group. May 9, 2013.

❖ Highest ranking in J.D. Power and Associates Member Satisfaction Study. J.D. Power and Associates. May 3, 2013.

❖ Worksite Innovation Award for KP Walk! and Platinum Fit-Friendly Companies Program Company Award. American Heart Association. May 2013.

❖ Pharmacy Quality Alliance's annual Quality Award for health plans achieving excellence in medication safety and quality. Pharmacy Quality Alliance. April 2, 2013.

❖ Guinness World Record for Most Colorectal Cancer Screenings. Guinness World Records. March 31, 2013.

❖ Highest rating on California's Annual Clinical Quality Report Card for overall quality of care for fifth consecutive year. Healthcare Quality Report Card from the California Office of the Patient Advocate. March 28, 2013.

❖ Highest rating in HMO category, which measures members' satisfaction with their total care and service. Healthcare Quality Report Card from the California Office of the Patient Advocate. March 28, 2013.

❖ Kaiser Permanente Health Plans Named eValue8's 2012 Top Performers, including awards for creativity and innovation in health care. National Business Coalition on Health. The March 11, 2013.

❖ Eisenberg Award for Patient Safety and Quality Efforts. The Joint Commission. March 2, 2013.

❖ Kaiser Permanente's Medicare Plans Earn Top NCQA Health Insurance Rankings. National Committee for Quality Assurance. 2012–2013.

2012
❖ Six eHealthcare Leadership Awards for the use of the Internet and technology to support the commitment to total health. Strategic Health Care Communications. November 30, 2012.

❖ Leapfrog Award for Kaiser Permanente Hospitals being among the safest in the nation. The Leapfrog Group. June 2012.

❖ Highest rating in the nation in 13 Medicare Measures. The 5-Star Star Quality rating system for Medicare Advantage Plans. Centers for Medicare and Medicaid Services (CMS). October 2012.

❖ Highest rating in the nation, Six 5-Star Medicare Health Plans. The 5-Star Star Quality Rating System for Medicare Advantage Plans. CMS. October 2012.

❖ Highest scores in the nation in 16 NCQA/HEDIS Effectiveness of Care Measures. National Committee for Quality Assurance (NCQA)/The Healthcare Effectiveness Data and Information Set (HEDIS). October, 2012.

❖ 20 hospitals ranked Top Performer in Quality. The Joint Commission. September 19, 2012.

❖ Leadership in Energy & Environmental Design (LEED) Platinum certification awarded to Napa Data Center. U.S. Green Building Design Council. July 2012.

❖ Highest in Customer Satisfaction among Mail-Order Pharmacies for fourth consecutive year. J.D. Power and Associates as. July 2012.

❖ Platinum Award for Best Employer for Healthy Lifestyles. National Business Group on Health. July 2012.

❖ Top 20 in Computerworld's 2012 List of 100 Best Places to Work in IT. International Data Group Network. July 2012

❖ Highest ranking in 2012 J.D. Power and Associates Employer Satisfaction Study for Second Year in a Row. J.D. Power and Associates. July 20, 2012.

❖ Leapfrog Awards. Kaiser Permanente Hospitals among the Safest in the Nation. The Leapfrog Group. July 2012.

❖ No. 1 in Customer Loyalty in the 2012 Satmetrix Net Promoter® Benchmark Study. The Net Promoter Company. March 2012.

❖ Laboratory of the year. The Medical Laboratory Observer. March 2012

❖ Stage 7 Awards. Healthcare Information and Management Systems Society (HIMSS). February, 2012.

2011

❖ Four eHealthcare Leadership Awards for the use of the Internet and technology to support the commitment to total health. Strategic Health Care Communications. December 7, 2011.

❖ Leapfrog Awards 18 Kaiser Permanente Hospitals as Top Hospitals for their outstanding success in such areas as infection rates, safety practices, mortality rates for common procedures and measures of efficiency. The Leapfrog Group. December 2011.

❖ Named No. 1 Green-IT Organization by Computerworld for excellence in IT practices that benefit the environment. International Data Group Network. October 2011.

❖ Recognized by J.D. Power and Associates as Highest in Customer Satisfaction among Mail-Order Pharmacies for Third Consecutive Year. J.D. Power & Associates. October 2011.

- ❖ 10 Kaiser Permanente Hospitals Honored as 'Top Performer' in Quality and Safety. The Joint Commission. September 2011.

- ❖ HIMSS Davies Award Presented for Organizational Excellence for Electronic Health Record Implementation. HIMSS Davies Award. September 2011.

- ❖ Pharmacy Quality Alliance's annual Quality Award for health plans achieving excellence in medication safety and quality. Pharmacy Quality Alliance. June 2011.

- ❖ U.S. News & World Report gives 13 Kaiser Permanente hospitals highest ranking for reputation, mortality, patient safety and other areas, including nurse staffing and technology. U.S. News & World Report. March 2011.

Endnotes for Charts

Chart 2.1: Getahun D, Strickland D, Zeiger RS, et al. Effect of Chorioamnionitis on Early Childhood Asthma. Arch Pediatr Adolesc Med. 2010;164(2):187-192. doi:10.1001/archpediatrics.2009.238.

Chart 2.2: Internal KP data. The Big Q Performance Metrics, 2012.

Chart 2.3: Internal KP data. The Big Q Performance Metrics, 2012.

Chart 2.4: Internal KP data. The Big Q Performance Metrics, 2012.

Chart 2.5: Internal KP data. The Big Q Performance Metrics, 2012.

Chart 2.6: US-SEER Sourced from SEER Cancer Statistics Review, 1975-2009 (Vintage 2009 populations), for invasive cases diagnosed 2002-2008. National Cancer Institute, Bethesda, MD, http://seer.cancer.gov/csr/1975_2009_pops09/, based on November 2011 SEER data submission, posted to the SEER web site, April 2012.

Chart 2.7: US-SEER Sourced from SEER Cancer Statistics Review, 1975-2009 (Vintage 2009 populations), for invasive cases diagnosed 2002-2008. National Cancer Institute, Bethesda, MD, http://seer.cancer.gov/csr/1975_2009_pops09/, based on November 2011 SEER data submission, posted to the SEER web site, April 2012.

Chart 2.8: US-SEER Sourced from SEER Cancer Statistics Review, 1975-2009 (Vintage 2009 populations), for invasive cases diagnosed 2002-2008. National Cancer Institute, Bethesda, MD, http://seer.cancer.gov/csr/1975_2009_pops09/, based on November 2011 SEER data submission, posted to the SEER web site, April 2012.

Chart 3.1: Internal KP data. The Big Q Performance Metrics, 2012.

Chart 4.1: Inpatient statin use predicts improved ischemic stroke discharge disposition. Kano O, Iwamoto K, Ikeda K, Iwasaki Y. Neurology. 2012 Dec 4; 79(23):2294.

Chart 4.2: Inpatient statin use predicts improved ischemic stroke discharge disposition. Kano O, Iwamoto K, Ikeda K, Iwasaki Y. Neurology. 2012 Dec 4; 79(23):2294.

Chart 4.3: US-SEER Sourced from SEER Cancer Statistics Review, 1975-2009 (Vintage 2009 populations), for invasive cases diagnosed 2002-2008. National Cancer Institute, Bethesda, MD, http://seer.cancer.gov/csr/1975_2009_pops09/, based on November 2011 SEER data submission, posted to the SEER web site, April 2012. Internal KP data. The Big Q Performance Metrics, 2012.

Chart 4.4: Internal KP data. The Big Q Performance Metrics, 2012.

Endnotes

1   Centers for Disease Control and Prevention. "Death in the United States, 2011." *NCHS Data Brief.* March 2013. http://www.cdc.gov/nchs/data/databriefs/db115.htm.

2   B. Smedley, A. Smith, and A. Nelson, editors. "Unequal Treatment: Confronting Racial and Ethnic Disparities in Health Care." *Institute of Medicine.* 2003.

3   Ibid.

4   S. Heffler and others. "Health Spending Projections for 2001–2011: The Latest Outlook." *Health Affairs.* 2002:21(2):207-218.

5   Ibid.

6   C. Weisse, P. Sorum, K. Sanders, and B Syat. "Do gender and race affect decisions about pain management?" *Journal of General Internal Medicine.* 2001:16(4):211-217

7   S. Broder-Fingert and others. "Racial and Ethnic Differences in Subspecialty Service Use by Children With Autism." *Pediatrics.* Published online June 17, 2013.
    http://pediatrics.aappublications.org/content/early/2013/06/12/peds.2012-3886.abstract.

8   Agency for Healthcare Research and Quality. "National Healthcare Quality Report 2012." May 2013.

9   "Black Women Have Higher Incidence of Multiple Sclerosis than White Women." *Kaiser Permanente News Center.* May 6, 2013.

http://xnet.kp.org/newscenter/pressreleases/nat/2013/050613-multiple-sclerosis-in-women.html.

10   D. Getahun and others. "Effect of Chorioamnionitis on Early Childhood Asthma." *Archives of Pediatric & Adolescent Medicine*. 2010:164(2):187-192.

11   Ibid.

12   Ibid

13   Ibid.

14   Centers for Disease Control and Prevention. "Cancer Screening – United States, 2010." *Morbidity and Mortality Weekly Report*. 2012:61(3).

15   Internal KP data: Kaiser Permanente's Interregional Cancer Incidence and Outcomes report. August 14, 2012.

16   Surveillance Epidemiology and End Results. "SEER State Fact Sheets: Colon and Rectum." http://seer.cancer.gov/statfacts/html/colorect.html#survival.

17   Centers for Disease Control. "Lung Cancer." http://www.cdc.gov/cancer/lung/.

18   Centers for Disease Control. "Chronic Diseases The Power to Prevent, The Call to Control: At A Glance 2009." http://www.cdc.gov/chronicdisease/resources/publications/AAG/chronic.htm.

19   M. O'Grady, P. John, and A. Winn. "Substantial Medicare Savings May Result If Insurers Cover 'Artificial Pancreas' Sooner For Diabetes Patients." *Health Affairs*. 2012:31(8):1822-1829.

20 Agency for Healthcare Research and Quality. "Diabetes Disparities Among Racial and Ethnic Minorities." http://www.ahrq.gov/research/findings/factsheets/diabetes/diabdisp/index.html.

21 Lancet Physical Activity Series Working Group. "Effect of physical inactivity on major non-communicable diseases worldwide: an analysis of burden of disease and life expectancy." *The Lancet*. 2012:380(9838):219-229.

22 Centers for Disease Control and Prevention. "FastStats - Exercise or Physical Activity." *National Center for Health Statistics*. http://www.cdc.gov/nchs/fastats/exercise.htm.

23 "F as in Fat: How Obesity Threatens America's Future." *Robert Wood Johnson Foundation Issue Report*. September 2012. OECD. "Health at a Glance 2011: OECD Indicators."

24 D. Lee and others. "Long-Term Effects of Changes in Cardiorespiratory Fitness and Body Mass Index on All-Cause and Cardiovascular Disease Mortality in Men." *Circulation*. 2011:124(23):2483-90.

25 American Diabetes Association. "Prediabetes FAQs." *Diabetes Basics*. http://www.diabetes.org/diabetes-basics/prevention/pre-diabetes/pre-diabetes-faqs.html.

26 United States Department of Health and Human Services. "HHS Targets Efforts on Diabetes." January 13, 2006. http://www.hhs.gov/news/factsheet/diabetes.html.

27 Arnold School of Public Health. "Study involved studying data from exams, treadmill tests at Cooper Clinic in Houston." *University of South Carolina*. March 23, 2009. http://www.sph.sc.edu/news/breastcancer.htm. K. Wolin and others. "Leisure-time physical activity patterns and risk of colon cancer in women."

International Journal of Cancer. 2007:121: 2776–2781. J. Antonelli and others. "Exercise and prostate cancer risk in a cohort of veterans undergoing prostate needle biopsy." *Journal of Urology.* 2009:182(5):2226-31. E. Giovannucci and others. "Physical Activity, Obesity, and Risk for Colon Cancer and Adenoma in Men." *Annals of Internal Medicine.* 1995:122:327-334.

28   J. Blumenthal et al.   "Effects of Exercise Training on Older Patients With Major Depression." *Archives of Internal Medicine.* 1999:159(19):2349-2356. J. Sieverdes and others. "Association between Leisure Time Physical Activity and Depressive Symptoms in Men." *Medicine and Science in Sports & Exercise.* 2012:44(2):260-265.

29   B. Smedley, A. Smith, and A. Nelson, editors. "Unequal Treatment: Confronting Racial and Ethnic Disparities in Health Care." *Institute of Medicine.* 2003.

30   Kaiser Permanente News Center. "Kaiser Foundation Hospitals and Health Plan Report Fiscal Year 2011 and Fourth Quarter Financial Results." February 10, 2012. http://xnet.kp.org/newscenter/pressreleases/nat/2012/021012q4yearendfinancials.html.

31   Kaiser Permanente. "2011 Annual Report." United States Census 2010. "Resident Population Data." http://www.census.gov/2010census/data/apportionment-pop-text.php.Central Intelligence Agency. "Country Comparison: Population." *The World Factbook.*   https://www.cia.gov/library/publications/the-world-factbook/rankorder/2119rank.html.

32   Kaiser Permanente News Center. "Kaiser Foundation Hospitals and Health Plan Report Fiscal Year 2011 and Fourth Quarter Financial Results." February 10, 2012. http://xnet.kp.org/newscenter/pressreleases/nat/2012/021012q4yearendfinancials.html.

33   E. Smith, A. Ziogas, H. Culver. "Delay in Surgical Treatment and Survival After Breast Cancer Diagnosis in Young Women by Race/Ethnicity." *JAMA Surgery*. 2013:148(6):516-523.

34   Ibid.

35   Centers for Disease Control and Prevention. "Cancer Screening – United States, 2010." *Morbidity and Mortality Weekly Report*. 2012:61(3).

36   A. Akincigil and others. "Racial and ethnic disparities in depression care in community-dwelling elderly in the United States." *American Journal of Public Health*. 2012:102(2):319-28.

37   G. Yan and others. "The associations between race and geographic area and quality-of-care indicators in patients approaching ESRD." *Clinical Journal of the American Society of Nephrology*. 2013:8(4):610-8.

38   Ibid.

39   C. Hebert and S. Bolen. "Best Practices in Achieving Equitable Care for Hypertension." http://betterhealthcleveland.org/BetterHealth/files/dd/dd57fc79-3ae1-4c21-b851-5d56b08eaaff.pdf .

40   Agency for Healthcare Research and Quality. *National Healthcare Quality Report 2012*. http://www.ahrq.gov/research/findings/nhqrdr.

41   Agency for Healthcare Research and Quality (AHRQ). *National Healthcare Quality Report 2012*. May 2013. http://www.ahrq.gov/research/findings/nhqrdr.

42   Ibid.

43   C. Weisse, P. Sorum, K. Sanders, and B Syat. "Do gender and race affect decisions about pain management?" *Journal of General Internal Medicine*. 2001:16(4):211–217.

44   Cram P, Bayman L, Popescu I, Vaughan-Sarrazin MS. (2009, November). Racial disparities in revascularization rates among patients with similar insurance coverage. *Journal of the National Medical Association*, 101(11):1132-9.

45   Agency for Healthcare Research and Quality. "National Healthcare Quality Report 2012." May 2013.

46   Ibid.

47   Centers for Disease Control and Prevention. "Diabetes Report Card 2012." http://www.cdc.gov/diabetes/pubs/pdf/DiabetesReportCard.pdf.

48   Ibid.

49   Centers for Disease Control and Prevention. HIV deaths by Race/Ethnicity Rate per 100,000 among selected population. 2010. http://gis.cdc.gov/GRASP/NCHHSTPAtlas/main.html.

50   Surveillance Epidemiology and End Results. "SEER State Fact Sheets: Cervix Uteri."
http://seer.cancer.gov/statfacts/html/cervix.html.

51   C. Weisse, P. Sorum, K. Sanders, and B Syat. "Do gender and race affect decisions about pain management?" *Journal of General Internal Medicine*. 2001:16(4):211-217

52   Centers for Disease Control and Prevention. "Diagnosed Diabetes by Race/Ethnicity, Sex, and Age." *Diabetes Data & Trends* http://www.cdc.gov/diabetes/statistics/prev/national/menuage.htm.

53 "Black Women Have Higher Incidence of Multiple Sclerosis than White Women." *Kaiser Permanente News Center*. May 6, 2013. http://xnet.kp.org/newscenter/pressreleases/nat/2013/050613-multiple-sclerosis-in-women.html.

54 American Diabetes Association. "Prediabetes FAQs." *Diabetes Basics*. http://www.diabetes.org/diabetes-basics/prevention/pre-diabetes/pre-diabetes-faqs.html.

55 Ibid.

56 D. Lee and others. "Long-Term Effects of Changes in Cardiorespiratory Fitness and Body Mass Index on All-Cause and Cardiovascular Disease Mortality in Men." *Circulation*. 2011:124(23):2483-90

57 G. Yan and others. "The associations between race and geographic area and quality-of-care indicators in patients approaching ESRD." *Clinical Journal of the American Society of Nephrology*. 2013:8(4):610-8.

58 S. Cohen and W. Yu. "The Concentration and Persistence in the Level of Health Expenditures over Time: Estimates for the U.S. Population, 2008–2009." *Agency for Healthcare Quality Statistical Brief #354*. January 2012. http://www.meps.ahrq.gov/mepsweb/data_files/publications/st354/stat354.pdf.

59 Centers for Disease Control. "Chronic Diseases The Power to Prevent, The Call to Control: At A Glance 2009." http://www.cdc.gov/chronicdisease/resources/publications/AAG/chronic.htm.

60 U.S. Department of Health and Human Services. "A Nation Free Of Disparities

In Health And Health Care." *HHS Action Plan to Reduce Racial and Ethnic Health Disparities.* http://minorityhealth.hhs.gov/npa/files/Plans/HHS/HHS_Plan_complete.pdf.

61   Kaiser Permanente Community Benefit. "Health Disparities: Notes and Insights." http://info.kaiserpermanente.org/communitybenefit/html/our_work/global/our_work_5_e.html.

62   Kaiser Family Foundation. "The Impact of Current State Medicaid Expansion Decision on Coverage by Race and Ethnicity." The Kaiser Commission on Medicaid and the Uninsured. July 2013. http://kaiserfamilyfoundation.files.wordpress.com/2013/06/8450-the-impact-of-current-state-medicaid-expansion-decisions.pdf

63   Ibid.

64   J. Appleby. "How Will the Health Law Impact Coverage for Immigrants?" *PBS Newshour.* October 12, 2012. http://www.pbs.org/newshour/rundown/2012/10/how-will-the-health-law-impact-coverage-for-immigrants.html.

65   Agency for Healthcare Research and Quality. "National Healthcare Quality Report 2012." May 2013.

66   B. Smedley, A. Smith, and A. Nelson, editors. "Unequal Treatment: Confronting Racial and Ethnic Disparities in Health Care." *Institute of Medicine.* 2003.

67   Kaiser Permanente. "About Kaiser Permanente: Fast Facts." http://xnet.kp.org/newscenter/aboutkp/fastfacts.html.

68   Ibid.

69   Internal KP data: Geographically Enriched Member Sociodemographic (GEMS) report. 2011.

70   Agency for Healthcare Research and Quality. "Disparities in Healthcare Quality Among Racial and Ethnic Minority Groups: Selected Findings From the 2010 National Healthcare Quality and Disparities Reports." March 2011.

71   Agency for Healthcare Research and Quality. "National Healthcare Quality Report 2012." May 2013.

72   Kaiser Permanente News Center. "Kaiser Foundation Hospitals and Health Plan Report Fiscal Year 2011 and Fourth Quarter Financial Results." February 10, 2012. http://xnet.kp.org/newscenter/pressreleases/nat/2012/021012q4yearendfinancials.html.

73   Kaiser Permanente. "About Kaiser Permanente: Fast Facts." http://xnet.kp.org/newscenter/aboutkp/fastfacts.html.

74   "Diversity & Inclusion Puts Kaiser Permanente on Top with Employees, Customers." *Diversity Inc.* http://www.diversityinc.com/diversity-events/what-makes-kaiser-permanente-no-1-for-diversity/.

75   Kaiser Permanente. "About Kaiser Permanente: Fast Facts." http://xnet.kp.org/newscenter/aboutkp/fastfacts.html.

76   Ibid.

77   "By the Numbers: Largest Group Practices." *Modern Healthcare.* September 26, 2011. http://www.modernhealthcare.com/article/20110926/DATA/110929995.

78   Internal Kaiser Permanente data. Daily Laboratory Tests Run and Viewed by Members. 2012.

79 Internal Kaiser Permanente data. & Estimated Daily Prescription Fill Volume. December 2012.

80 Kaiser Permanente. "2011 Annual Report." United States Census 2010. "Resident Population Data." http://www.census.gov/2010census/data/apportionment-pop-text.php. Central Intelligence Agency. "Country Comparison: Population." *The World Factbook.* https://www.cia.gov/library/publications/the-world-factbook/rankorder/2119rank.html.

81 Kaiser Permanente. "About Kaiser Permanente: Fast Facts." http://xnet.kp.org/newscenter/aboutkp/fastfacts.html.

82 B. Snyder. "How Kaiser bet $4 billion on electronic health records -- and won." *InfoWorld.com.* May 2, 2013. http://www.infoworld.com/d/the-industry-standard/how-kaiser-bet-4-billion-electronic-health-records-and-won-217731.

83 "Diversity & Inclusion Puts Kaiser Permanente on Top with Employees, Customers." *Diversity Inc.* http://www.diversityinc.com/diversity-events/what-makes-kaiser-permanente-no-1-for-diversity/.

84 Kaiser Permanente. "Executive Biographies." *About KP.* http://xnet.kp.org/newscenter/aboutkp/bios/index.html.

85 Ibid.

86 Kaiser Permanente News Center. "Kaiser Permanente Leads the Nation with Six 5-Star Medicare Health Plans." October 15, 2012. http://xnet.kp.org/newscenter/pressreleases/nat/2012/101512_medicare_stars_final.html

87 Ibid.

88 Ibid.

89   J.D. Power. "2012 U.S. Member Health Plan Study." March 12, 2012. http://www.jdpower.com/content/press-release/8UhZWgn/2012-u-s-member-health-plan-study.htm.

90 "About The Score – Hospital Safety Score." *Hospital Safety Score*. http://www.hospitalsafetyscore.org/about-the-score.

91   Kaiser Permanente News Center. "Kaiser Permanente Hospitals Rated Among Safest in the Nation." May 9, 2013. http://xnet.kp.org/newscenter/pressreleases/nat/2013/050913-leapfrog-top-hospitals.html.

92   The Joint Commission. "2012 John M. Eisenberg Patient Safety and Quality Award Recipients Announced." February 6, 2013.

93   HIMSS Analytics. "Stage 7 Hospitals." http://www.himssanalytics.org/hc_providers/stage7Hospitals.asp.

94   Uptime Institute. "Green Enterprise IT Awards Honorees." *Symposium Uptime Institute*. http://symposium.uptimeinstitute.com/geit-awards/1840-geit-awards-honorees-all.

95   http://xnet.kp.org/newscenter/pressreleases/nat/2013/052213-leed-gold-building-practices.html

96   Satmetrix. "USAA, Amazon.com, Costco, Virgin America, Apple, Trader Joe's & Wegmans, Among the Highest in Customer Loyalty in the 2012 Satmetrix Net Promoter Benchmark Study." March 14, 2012. http://www.satmetrix.com/company/press-and-news/pr-archive/pr20120314/.

97   Agency for Healthcare Research and Quality. "Race, Ethnicity, and Language Data: Standardization for Health Care Quality Improvement, Appendix E, Table E-1." http://www.ahrq.gov/legacy/research/iomracereport/reldataaptabe1.htm.

98 "Black Women Have Higher Incidence of Multiple Sclerosis than White Women." *Kaiser Permanente News Center*. May 6, 2013. http://xnet.kp.org/newscenter/pressreleases/nat/2013/050613-multiple-sclerosis-in-women.html.

99 D. Getahun and others. "Effect of Chorioamnionitis on Early Childhood Asthma." *Archives of Pediatric & Adolescent Medicine*. 2010:164(2):187-192.

100 National Committee for Quality Assurance. "Focus on Obesity and on Medicare Plan Improvement." *The State of Health Care Quality 2012*. October 2012.

101 Internal KP data.

102 Ibid.

103 Ibid.

104 S. Omer and others. "Vaccine Refusal, Mandatory Immunization, and the Risks of Vaccine-Preventable Diseases." *New England Journal of Medicine*. 2009:360:1981-1988.

105 Institute of Medicine. "Immunization Safety Review: Vaccines and Autism. Executive Summary." 2004. http://www.iom.edu/Reports/2004/Immunization-Safety-Review-Vaccines-and-Autism.aspx.

106 Surveillance Epidemiology and End Results. "SEER State Fact Sheets: Colon and Rectum." http://seer.cancer.gov/statfacts/html/colorect.html#survival.

107 Internal KP data: Kaiser Permanente's Interregional Cancer Incidence and Outcomes Report. August 14, 2012.

108 Surveillance Epidemiology and End Results. "SEER State Fact Sheets: Colon and Rectum." http://seer.cancer.gov/statfacts/html/colorect.html#survival.

109 Internal KP data: Kaiser Permanente's Interregional Cancer Incidence and Outcomes Report. August 14, 2012.

110 Surveillance Epidemiology and End Results. "SEER State Fact Sheets: Breast." http://seer.cancer.gov/statfacts/html/breast.html#survival.

111 Internal KP data: Kaiser Permanente's Interregional Cancer Incidence and Outcomes Report. August 14, 2012.

112 Surveillance Epidemiology and End Results. "SEER State Fact Sheets: Breast." http://seer.cancer.gov/statfacts/html/breast.html#survival.

113 B. Smedley, A. Smith, and A. Nelson, editors. "Unequal Treatment: Confronting Racial and Ethnic Disparities in Health Care." *Institute of Medicine.* 2003.

114 Kaiser Permanente. "Meeting HIV/AIDS Workforce Challenges With Multidisciplinary Care Teams." *Institute for Health Policy.* 2012. http://www.kpihp.org/wp-content/uploads/2012/06/KPStories-v1-no5-HIV_AIDS-FINAL.pdf.

115 Kaiser Permanente. "Take the HIV Challenge." http://info.kaiserpermanente.org/communitybenefit/html/our_work/global/hivchallenge/hiv_challenge.html.

116 Kaiser Permanente Community Benefit. "Health Disparities: Notes and Insights." http://info.kaiserpermanente.org/communitybenefit/html/our_work/global/our_work_5_e.html.

117 Centers for Disease Control. "Chronic Diseases The Power to Prevent, The Call to Control: At A Glance 2009." http://www.cdc. gov/chronicdisease/resources/publications/AAG/chronic.htm. G. Anderson. "Chronic Care: Making the Case for Ongoing Care." *Robert Wood Johnson Foundation*. February 2010. www.rwjf.org/pr/product. jsp?id=50968.

118 C. Schoen and others. "A Survey of Primary Care Doctors in Ten Countries Shows Progress in Use of Health Information Technology, Less in Other Areas." Health Affairs Web First. November 15, 2012.

119 G. Anderson. "Chronic Care: Making the Case for Ongoing Care." Robert Wood Johnson Foundation. February 2010. www. rwjf.org/pr/product.jsp?id=50968.

120 Agency for Healthcare Quality and Research. "Patient Centered Medical Home Resource Center." http://www.pcmh. ahrq.gov/portal/server.pt/community/pcmh__home/1483.

121 Agency for Healthcare Quality and Research. "Coordinating Care for Adults With Complex Care Needs in the Patient-Centered Medical Home: Challenges and Solutions." January 2012.

122 M. Nielsen and others. "Benefits of Implementing the Primary Care Patient-Centered Medical Home: A Review of Cost & Quality Results 2012." *Patient-Centered Primary Care Collaborative*. 2012.

123 Agency for Healthcare Research and Quality. "Patient Centered Medical Home Resource Center." http://www.pcmh. ahrq.gov/portal/server.pt/community/pcmh__home/1483.

124 Centers for Disease Control. "Chronic Diseases The Power to Prevent, The Call to Control: At A Glance 2009." http://www.

cdc.gov/chronicdisease/resources/publications/AAG/chronic.
htm.

125 U.S. Department of Health and Human Services. "A Nation Free Of Disparities
In Health And Health Care." *HHS Action Plan to Reduce Racial and Ethnic Health Disparities.* http://minorityhealth.hhs.gov/npa/ files/Plans/HHS/HHS_Plan_complete.pdf.

126 E. Woods and others. "Community Asthma Initiative: Evaluation of a Quality Improvement Program for Comprehensive Asthma Care." *Pediatrics.* 2012:129(3):465-472.

127 N. Pheatt, R. Brindis, and E. Levin. "Putting Heart Disease Guidelines into Practice: Kaiser Permanente Leads the Way." The Permanente Journal. 2003:7(1):18-23.

128 E. Woods and others. "Community Asthma Initiative: Evaluation of a Quality Improvement Program for Comprehensive Asthma Care." *Pediatrics.* 2012:129(3):465-472.

129 N. Pheatt, R. Brindis, and E. Levin. "Putting Heart Disease Guidelines into Practice: Kaiser Permanente Leads the Way." The Permanente Journal. 2003:7(1):18-23.

130 N. Pheatt, R. Brindis, and E. Levin. "Putting Heart Disease Guidelines into Practice: Kaiser Permanente Leads the Way." *The Permanente Journal.* 2003:7(1):18-23. Editorial. "Simple Treatments, Ignored." *New York Times.* September 8, 2012. http://www.nytimes. com/2012/09/09/opinion/sunday/simple-treatments-ignored. html?_r=2&.

131 S. Heffler and others. "Health Spending Projections for 2001–2011: The Latest Outlook." Health Affairs. 2002:21(2):207-218.

132   E.   Emanuel.   "Spending   More   Doesn't   Make Us   Healthier."   New   York   Times.   October   27,   2011. http://opinionator.blogs.nytimes.com/2011/10/27/ spending-more-doesnt-make-us-healthier/?_r=0.

133 B. Smedley, A. Smith, and A. Nelson, editors. "Unequal Treatment: Confronting Racial and Ethnic Disparities in Health Care." Institute of Medicine. 2003.

134 M. Eber, R. Laxminarayan, E. Perencevich, and A. Malani. "Clinical and Economic Outcomes Attributable to Health Care–Associated Sepsis and Pneumonia." Archives of Internal Medicine. 2010:170(4): 347-353.

135 A. Haider and others. "Association Between Hospitals Caring for a Disproportionately High Percentage of Minority Trauma Patients and Increased Mortality." Archives of Surgery. 2012:147(1):63-70.

136 National Institute of General Medical Sciences. "Sepsis Fact Sheet." November 2012. http://www.nigms.nih.gov/Education/ factsheet_sepsis.htm.

137 National Institute of General Medical Sciences. "Sepsis Fact Sheet." November 2012. http://www.nigms.nih.gov/Education/ factsheet_sepsis.htm.

138 California Office of Statewide Health Planning and Development "In-Hospital Mortality, 2006." OSHPD Research Brief. November 2008.

139 M. Raghavan and P. Marik. "Management of sepsis during the early 'golden hours.'" The Journal of Emergency Medicine. 2006: 31(2):185 199.

140 Kaiser Permanente. "Take the HIV Challenge." http:// info.kaiserpermanente.org/communitybenefit/html/our_work/ global/hivchallenge/hiv_challenge.html.

141 Kaiser Permanente. "Reducing Pressure Ulcers in Kaiser Foundation Hospitals." *Measuring Patient Safety in our Hospitals.* May 2012. https://healthy.kaiserpermanente.org/static/health/ pdfs/quality_and_safety/multi/multi_pressure_ulcers.pdf.

142 National Quality Measures Clearinghouse. "Pressure ulcer prevention and treatment protocol: percentage of inpatients with pressure ulcers whose medical record contains documentation of a partial wound assessment with every dressing change." *Agency for Healthcare Research and Quality.* http://qualitymeasures.ahrq.gov/ content.aspx?id=36735.

143 Ibid.

144 Kaiser Permanente. "Reducing Pressure Ulcers in Kaiser Foundation Hospitals." *Measuring Patient Safety in our Hospitals.* May 2012. https://healthy.kaiserpermanente.org/static/health/ pdfs/quality_and_safety/multi/multi_pressure_ulcers.pdf.

145 KP internal data on Nursing SKKIN Bundle and HEROES program work.

146 D. Cosgrove and others. "A CEO Checklist for High-Value Health Care." *Institute of Medicine Discussion Paper.* June 5, 2012. http://www.iom.edu/Global/Perspectives/2012/CEOChecklist. aspx.

147 D. Cosgrove and others. "A CEO Checklist for High-Value Health Care." *Institute of Medicine Discussion Paper.* June 5, 2012. http://www.iom.edu/Global/Perspectives/2012/ CEOChecklist.aspx.

KP internal data: Nursing SKKIN Bundle and HEROES program work.

148 Kaiser Permanente News Center. "Healthy Bones Program Reduces Hip Fractures by 37 Percent, Kaiser Permanente Study Finds." November 4, 2008. http://xnet.kp.org/newscenter/press-releases/nat/2008/110408healthybones.html

149 R. Dell, D. Greene, S. Schelkun, and K. Williams. "Osteoporosis Disease Management: The Role of the Orthopedic Surgeon." *The Journal of Bone & Joint Surgery.* 2008:90(4):188-194.

150 International Federation of Health Plans. "2011 Comparative Price Report Medical and Hospital Fees by Country." http://www.ifhp.com/documents/2011iFHPPriceReportGraphs_version3.pdf.

151 Kaiser Permanente. "2011 Annual Report."

152 B. Snyder. "How Kaiser bet $4 billion on electronic health records -- and won." *InfoWorld.com.* May 2, 2013. http://www.infoworld.com/d/the-industry-standard/how-kaiser-bet-4-billion-electronic-health-records-and-won-217731.

153 Editorial. "Simple Treatments, Ignored." *New York Times.* September 8, 2012. http://www.nytimes.com/2012/09/09/opinion/sunday/simple-treatments-ignored.html?_r=2&.

154 "NIH Public Access Policy Does Not Affect U.S. Copyright Law." *Association of Research Libraries.* July 2008. http://www.sparc.arl.org/bm~doc/nihpolicy_copyright_july2008.pdf.

155 B. Smedley, A. Smith, and A. Nelson, editors. "Unequal Treatment: Confronting Racial and Ethnic Disparities in Health Care." *Institute of Medicine.* 2003.

156 Institute of Medicine Roundtable on Evidence-Based Medicine. "Leadership Commitments to Improve Value in Healthcare: Finding Common Ground: Workshop Summary." *National Academies Press.* 2009. http://www.ncbi.nlm.nih.gov/books/NBK52847/.

157 R. Hoban. "Nurses Embrace Evidence in Their Daily Practice." *North Carolina Health News.* September 26, 2012. http://www.northcarolinahealthnews.org/2012/09/26/nurses-embrace-evidence-in-their-daily-practice/.

158 S. Young and others. "Sharing Clinical Knowledge." *Kaiser Permanente Care Management Institute.* July 10, 2012. http://www.iom.edu/~/media/Files/Activity%20Files/Quality/VSRT/IC%20Meeting%20Docs/ICD%2007-10-12/Scott%20Young.pdf.

159 Internal KP data.

160 S. Young and others. "Sharing Clinical Knowledge." *Kaiser Permanente Care Management Institute.* July 10, 2012. http://www.iom.edu/~/media/Files/Activity%20Files/Quality/VSRT/IC%20Meeting%20Docs/ICD%2007-10-12/Scott%20Young.pdf.

161 *A.C. Flint and others.* "Inpatient Statin use Predicts Improved Ischemic Stroke Discharge Disposition." *Neurology.* 2012:78(21):1678-1683.

162 Ibid.

163 Ibid.

164 Ibid.

165 "NIH Public Access Policy Does Not Affect U.S. Copyright Law." *Association of Research Libraries.* July 2008. http://www.sparc.arl.org/bm~doc/nihpolicy_copyright_july2008.pdf.

166 Kaiser Permanente. "About Kaiser Permanente: Fast Facts." http://xnet.kp.org/newscenter/aboutkp/fastfacts.html.

167 Kaiser Permanente. "2011 Annual Report." Kaiser Permanente News Center. "Integrated Health Care Delivery System and Electronic Health Records Support Medication Adherence." September 6, 2011. http://xnet.kp.org/newscenter/pressreleases/nat/2011/090611medicationadherence.html. http://xnet.kp.org/newscenter/annualreport.

168 Ibid.

169 Kaiser Permanente. "2011 Annual Report."

170 S. Machlin and K. Carper. "Expenses for Office-Based Physician Visits by Specialty, 2004." *MEPS Statistical Brief #166*. March 2007.

171 Kaiser Permanente. "Reducing Pressure Ulcers in Kaiser Foundation Hospitals." *Measuring Patient Safety in our Hospitals.* May 2012. https://healthy.kaiserpermanente.org/static/health/pdfs/quality_and_safety/multi/multi_pressure_ulcers.pdf.

172 Kaiser Permanente News Center. "Celebrating Winning the Battle Against Pressure Ulcers." February 15, 2013. http://xnet.kp.org/newscenter/ceoletters/2013/021513_ulcers.html.

173 M. Eber, R. Laxminarayan, E. Perencevich, and A. Malani. "Clinical and Economic Outcomes Attributable to Health Care–Associated Sepsis and Pneumonia." *Archives of Internal Medicine*. 2010:170(4): 347-353.

174 National Cancer Insitute. Suveillance, Epidemiology, and End Results. SEER stat Fact Sheets: http://seer.cancer.gov/statfacts/html/breast.html#survival; Internal KP data: Kaiser

Permanente's Interregional Cancer Incidence and Outcomes report, August 14, 2012.

175 Healthgrades. "America's Best Hospitals 2013: Navigating Variability in Hospital Quality." 2013.
http://hg-article-center.s3-website-us-east-1.amazonaws.com/a9/7b/2954b09f4822bb81649a1f06a6cf/healthgrades-americas-best-hospitals-report-2013.pdf.

176 California Office of Statewide Health Planning and Development. "The California Report on Coronary Artery Bypass Graft Surgery, 2009 Hospital Data." April 2012.

177 National Institute of General Medical Sciences. "Sepsis Fact Sheet." November 2012. http://www.nigms.nih.gov/Education/factsheet_sepsis.htm.

178 Health Behavior News Service. "Predominately Black Hospitals Provide Poor Trauma Care." May 16, 2013. http://www.newswise.com/articles/predominately-black-hospitals-provide-poor-trauma-care.

179 Kaiser Permanente. "2011 Annual Report."

180 Kaiser Permanente. "2011 Annual Report." United States Census 2010. "Resident Population Data." http://www.census.gov/2010census/data/apportionment-pop-text.php. Central Intelligence Agency. "Country Comparison: Population." *The World Factbook*. https://www.cia.gov/library/publications/the-world-factbook/rankorder/2119rank.html.

181 Internal KP data. Geographically Enriched Member Sociodemographics (GEMS) reort. 2011; Agency for Healthcare Research and Quality. "Disparities in Healthcare Quality Among Racial and Ethnic Minority Groups: Selected Findings From the 2010 National Healthcare Quality and Disparities Reports." March 2011.

182 Internal KP data. Geographically Enriched Member Sociodemographics (GEMS) reort. 2011.

183 "Diversity & Inclusion Puts Kaiser Permanente on Top with Employees, Customers." *Diversity Inc.* http://www.diversityinc.com/diversity-events/what-makes-kaiser-permanente-no-1-for-diversity/.

184 Kaiser Permanente. "Executive Biographies." *About KP.* http://xnet.kp.org/newscenter/aboutkp/bios/index.html.

185 A. Chadwick. "Remembering Tuskegee Syphilis Study Still Provokes Disbelief, Sadness." *National Public Radio.* July 2002. http://www.npr.org/programs/morning/features/2002/jul/tuskegee/.

186 S. Broder-Fingert and others. "Racial and Ethnic Differences in Subspecialty Service Use by Children With Autism." *Pediatrics.* Published online June 17, 2013.
http://pediatrics.aappublications.org/content/early/2013/06/12/peds.2012-3886.abstract.

187 "The DiversityInc Top 50 Companies for Diversity." *Diversity Inc.* http://www.diversityinc.com/the-diversityinc-top-50-companies-for-diversity-2013/.

188 Kaiser Permanente News Center. "Kaiser Permanente Receives Inaugural Honor from Diversity MBA Magazine." April 30, 2012. http://xnet.kp.org/newscenter/pressreleases/nat/2012/043012diversitymba.html.

189 "100 Best Places to Work in IT 2012." *ComputerWorld.* http://www.computerworld.com/spring/bp/detail/917.

190 Kaiser Permanente News Center. "Kaiser Permanente's Latino Employee Resource Group Honored as Among Top in the

Nation by U.S. Hispanic Chamber of Commerce." September 24, 2012. http://xnet.kp.org/newscenter/pressreleases/nat/2012/092412_latino_association_honored.html.

191 Health Behavior NewsService. "Predominately Black Hospitals Provide Poor Trauma Care." May 16, 2013. http://www.newswise.com/articles/predominately-black-hospitals-provide-poor-trauma-care.

192 Centers for Disease Control and Prevention. "Death in the United States, 2011." *NCHS Data Brief.* March 2013. http://www.cdc.gov/nchs/data/databriefs/db115.htm.